OUR WORLD RUNS ON ELECTRICITY. HAVE YOU ASKED YOURSELF . . .

✦ Do I live too close to power lines? Will they cause cancer in my children?

✦ Can cellular phones really cause brain cancer?

✦ How can I identify EMF and EMR sources at home and at work?

✦ Are my hair dryer and toaster dangerous?

✦ Is it safe to sleep under an electric blanket?

✦ Is it safe for my children to play video games?

✦ Am I at risk when I use my computer at work?

✦ How can I get action and answers from my electric utility company?

✦ Who in the federal government is responsible for EMF and EMR?

✦ Why can't I get straight answers when I ask questions about EMF and EMR?

✦ Who is going to pay for solutions to the EMF and EMR problem?

Get the answers to these questions and scores more in . . .

THE EMF BOOK
What You Need to Know About Electromagnetic Fields, Electromagnetic Radiation, and Your Health

Turn this page for praise on THE EMF BOOK

P9-CCK-911

"An indispensable guide . . . a practical and user-friendly book that should be required reading for anyone needing more information about EMFs—and that includes all of us."

—Joel Shufro, executive director, New York Committee for Occupational Safety and Health

"THE EMF BOOK is a valuable resource for anyone who wants a comprehensive introduction to this emerging but uncertain area of scientific activity."

—Dr. Robert B. Goldberg, Information Ventures, Inc.

"A terrific reference manual! It fills a great void for people trying to come to grips with the issue . . . and is both educational and practical. This book provides a much needed single source of information about EM fields and their possible hazards."

—Dottie English, board member, National EMR Alliance

"Mr. Pinsky has taken a complicated, vital subject and made it accessible . . . readable, entertaining, and above all, balanced. The subject needs the respect which Mr. Pinsky affords it."

—Michael Hiles, president and CEO, Norad Corporation

✦ ✦ ✦

"Here is a visionary book that will be seen as amazingly on target . . . practical, balanced, well informed, I welcome THE EMF BOOK as must reading on the number one environmental issue in America."

—George S. Lechter, Safe Technologies Corporation

THE EMF BOOK

What You Should Know About Electromagnetic Fields, Electromagnetic Radiation, and Your Health

MARK A. PINSKY

WARNER BOOKS

A Time Warner Company

Copyright © 1995 by Mark A. Pinsky

All rights reserved.

Warner Books, Inc., 1271 Avenue of the Americas, New York, NY 10020

 A Time Warner Company

Printed in the United States of America

First Printing: January 1995

10 9 8 7 6 5 4 3 2 1

Library of Congress Cataloging-in-Publication Data

Pinsky, Mark A.
   The EMF book : what you should know about electromagnetic fields, electromagnetic radiation, and your health / Mark A. Pinsky.
      p.   cm.
   Includes bibliographical references and index.
   ISBN 0-446-67004-9
   1. electromagnetic fields—Health aspects.   2. Electromagnetic fields—Safety measures.   3. Electromagnetic fields—Government policy—United States.   I. Title.
RA569-3.P54   1995
363.18'9—dc20   94-21776
                                                   CIP

Book design by H. Roberts
Cover design by Diane Luger
Cover photograph by Lester Lefkowitz/Tony Stone Images

To my family

ACKNOWLEDGEMENTS

MANY PEOPLE HAVE CONTRIBUTED TO THIS BOOK IN SMALL AND big ways. For particular help and support in researching and writing, my appreciation goes to Dan Dasho, Robert Goldberg, Tina Irvin, Colleen Kapklein, Ed Leeper, Jennifer Paget, Dr. Linda Pinsky, Karl Riley, Jerry Sontag, and Dave Weiss.

I have strived to make this book precise and accurate. In simplifying complex scientific information, I may have condensed some data in pursuit of clarity. This is unfortunate but unavoidable.

CONTENTS

INTRODUCTION

THIS BOOK IS ABOUT ELECTROMAGNETIC FIELDS (EM FIELDS) AND electromagnetic radiation (EM radiation)—two forms of energy. Everyone who lives or works near electronic devices or who uses electricity is exposed to one or the other, or to both. EM fields and EM radiation are present almost everywhere you are.

Not long ago I made a list of the ways my family and I are exposed. We live in a suburban community, and so our experience is similar to millions of other people's. We have power distribution wires strung on telephone poles along the edge of our property, and feeder wires bring power from the distribution line to our house. My wife and I have an electric bedside alarm clock, and my son has a lamp clipped to his bunk bed. Our stove is electric, and in our kitchen there is a microwave oven, a mixer, a coffeemaker, a washing machine, a dishwasher, and two small fluorescent lights. We have two television sets, one "boom box" radio, and a component stereo. Our forty-five-year-old house has metal (as opposed to plastic) plumbing, which can conduct electricity. Though we cannot see the wiring in the walls, the electrical outlets every ten to fifteen feet show us the path electricity takes. My son's playroom, located directly below the master bedroom, has a ceiling fan.

In my office, I use both a desktop and a laptop computer. My desk lamp uses a halogen bulb, and the heavy base contains a transformer that, like all transformers, emits relatively high EM field levels. The electric power feeder line runs along the outside wall of my office, though the "drop-off point" is in the basement of the building, two stories down. The photocopier and laser printer—both known to put out strong EM fields—are in a far, outside corner of the second office in my suite.

My son's day-care center has fewer exposure sources inside, but 200 feet away is a large, green metal structure that contains a transformer serving not only the day-care building but also the neighboring hospital. Visible from the day-care center is an electric power transmission line, the type suspended from tall metal towers. It is too far from the day-care center to concern me, but nearby it cuts across an elementary school yard and within fifty feet of one side of the school. It also passes near a residential development.

Driving in my community, I pass industrial buildings with small lattice metal towers supporting radio transmitters for local delivery systems. Along the way, I see microwave relay dishes—they look a little like gray kettledrums on their sides.

I have made many choices to reduce my EM field and EM radiation exposures. I do not use cellular or cordless phones, except in emergencies. I used a meter to measure EM fields and EM radiation to identify the areas in my home where the levels were highest, and I made some changes. My wife and I placed my son's crib, and later his bed, in the area in his room where EM fields were lowest. Instead of a wireless room monitor, we used an intercom with a wire. Our television sets are located so that they back against outside walls, since the highest EM radiation levels occur at the back and on the sides. For the same reason, I set up my computers so that exposures are minimal under normal circumstances. The copier and laser printer are in a far corner, away from desks and common work areas. The halogen lamp is pushed as far back on the desk as possible. The wires bringing electricity to my office building are new, bundled wires that are known to produce significantly lower EM field levels than older wiring systems. Though I did not take measurements in the office, I used a simple experiment to determine that the EM field levels were low. I placed a computer monitor along the wall near the bundled wires to see whether the image on the screen was distorted in any way, a problem that occurs when a strong field is present. The image was unaffected.

In our kitchen we put our microwave oven on top of the refrigerator, as far as possible from my son, and we make a point of keeping our distance while it operates. We usually run the dishwasher and washing machine only when we are in other rooms or out of the house. The electric stove is hard to avoid when we're cooking. We turn the fluorescent lights on only when we really need them.

We never leave the ceiling fan running while my wife and I are in our bedroom. When I took measurements in and around our home, I looked for—and fortunately did not find—evidence of high EM fields from electricity running along the metal plumbing.

While generally reassuring, my survey raised a few concerns, particularly the pervasiveness of EM field and EM radiation sources. Every day I notice a potential emissons source that I had overlooked previously. At the same time, everywhere I go I scan for sources to try to identify practical ways to reduce exposures. Almost always the solutions are clear and simple.

If you have heard about EM *fields*, most likely it was in conjunction with power lines. Scientific research has linked power lines with childhood cancer, some types of adult cancer, and other health disorders. For the past fifteen years, public interest in EM fields has grown steadily, encompassing not only power lines but also the wiring in our homes, the computers we use at work and at home, appliances such as hair dryers and razors that make our lives easier, and other electrical devices.

EM *radiation*, a broad category that includes everything from microwaves to radio broadcasts to cellular phone signals, is similar to EM fields in many respects but different in key ways (see Chapter 4). Scientists have been probing possible health effects for more than fifty years, and have found evidence of hazards almost from the start. In the mid-1970s, briefly, pockets of public concern developed, most often over plans to build new satellite communications facilities or to increase the size or power of a television or radio transmitter. More recently, claims that police radar devices cause cancer and that cellular phones may do the same have catapulted EM radiation back into the public eye.

In most public discussions, EM fields are known as EMFs, while EM radiation is called nonionizing radiation, nonionizing electromagnetic radiation, or sometimes just microwave or radiofrequency radiation. This book uses *EM fields* and *EM radiation* to reduce confusion.

The EMF Book explains in a straightforward way the scientific research that has prompted concern about EM field and EM radiation health effects, tells you how to look for EM field and EM radiation sources, and explains what you can do to reduce your exposures.

You can take steps to protect yourself and your family without knowing every scientific detail about EM fields and EM radiation. I have tried to provide pertinent information in a balanced way so that you can reach your own conclusions with confidence. Most of the steps you can take are fairly simple and inexpensive—ranging from rewiring to increasing distances between EM field and radiation sources and people. Reducing exposures while we wait for more definitive answers—and it will be a long wait—need not always be expensive, intrusive, or difficult. Engineers have found myriad low-cost and no-cost ways to reduce exposures in public places. In some instances, it is as simple as flipping a switch.

Not all situations are simple, however. Some readers may face unusual exposure conditions or be unable to identify the sources of the exposures due to a complexity of wiring systems or unknown sources. Readers who find themselves at odds with their electric utility, a private company, public officials, or their employers need to know what precedents exist. There is an extensive history of legal disputes, citizen action to oppose legislative debates, and regulatory rulings that have served as de facto public policy. *The EMF Book* recounts the major decisions and describes how a diverse set of public officials, citizens, and companies have addressed health concerns.

Ultimately, this book should be used as a resource and a reference. Section 4 includes a comprehensive guide to key research, a glossary you can refer to for scientific terminology, and suggestions for further reading.

Too many times over the past decade, people who simply want to find out what EM fields and EM radiation are, whether they pose a hazard, and how to protect themselves and their loved ones have had to start from scratch. Until now there has been no comprehensive, clear, reliable, and affordable handbook. It is to meet these needs that I wrote *The EMF Book*.

Mark A. Pinsky
Lower Makefield, PA

Understanding EM Fields and EM Radiation

CHAPTER 1

GRAPPLING WITH
EM FIELD AND
EM RADIATION
HEALTH EFFECTS

DOTTIE ENGLISH AND HER HUSBAND, FRANK, ARE UNLIKELY activists. "Neither Frank nor I were ever involved in community issues before EM fields," she explains. "We worked all day, came home, and in some cases we hardly even knew our neighbors." Now in her mid-fifties, Dottie English is a businesswoman who speaks softly and calmly, dresses conservatively, exercises extreme restraint in her statements, and always makes her points carefully and logically. That, one utility official explained, is what made her a threat.

Many of the people concerned about EM fields and EM radiation have young children, and most, like Dottie English, have no history of activism. Some fear for their children, some for themselves, some for their property values. "Concern about the research on kids and cancer really sent people through the roof," English says.

Dottie led a quiet, suburban life until 1990, when she learned that Philadelphia Electric Company (PECO) was installing a new electric power transmission line along an abandoned railroad track behind their home in upper Southampton, Pennsylvania. One of the company's workers told the Englishes that he would be concerned about the EM fields the line would emit if he were them. A few weeks later at a public meeting, a utility spokesman announced that the projected EM field levels in the yards next to the proposed line would be nothing to worry about, even though he said the levels would be about 20 milligauss. By then, the Englishes knew on the basis of news stories that this was ten times as high as the exposure levels that several studies had linked to cancer in children.

"The electric company brought the opposition on itself," Dottie English believes. "They were telling us there was no reason to be concerned before we even knew anything about the transmission line." The utility told them not to discuss the line with their neighbors and not to ask questions at local municipal meetings.

Within a month the Englishes had plunged into the research data and found themselves part of a burgeoning international network of people in similar situations. What they were reading and hearing worried them. "Once you start looking at the volume of research and the length of time it has been around, it starts to look like someone wanted to keep us from the facts," she says.

They organized a local group, Parents Against an UnSafe Environment (PAUSE), forced the state Public Utility Commission (PUC) to reopen its deliberations on the planned power line, and forced Pennsylvania's public officials to take their first serious look at EM fields, just as officials in dozens of other states were doing. Although they eventually lost their challenge when the PUC refused to hear testimony from scientists supporting their claims, they raised awareness of an important issue.

At home, Dottie and Frank made changes they thought would help protect them. They rearranged furniture, lights, and their television set to reduce their exposures based on what they had learned. They decided to stay away from their dishwasher and microwave oven when they were in use. "We didn't stop using electricity. It's a vital part of our life," she notes. Some neighbors took more severe actions. One family threw away its microwave oven, and several stopped using many other appliances.

A growing number of people who have closely evaluated the EM field and EM radiation research have found ways to reduce exposure levels. Granger Morgan, a prominent researcher at Carnegie Mellon University in Pittsburgh, Pennsylvania, moved his son's bed across the room, stopped using electric blankets, and shifted electric bedside clocks away from the beds. Diane Allen, a television reporter who investigated the EM field controversy, revealed at a congressional hearing that her reporting led her to bury the electric wires that bring power to her home. The lead author of a U.S. Environmental Protection Agency report recommending that EM fields be classified as "probable human carcinogens" and that EM radiation be labeled "possible human carcinogens" put away his electric razor, and measured levels in his home to see if there were exposure conditions of concern.

Like the Englishes, some people have organized community groups to raise awareness about EM fields and EM radiation and, in some instances, to oppose new or existing sources of emissions. People have organized in places as diverse as suburban New Jersey, rural Michigan, and New York City. Some have quit their jobs to press EM field or EM radiation issues, and some have sold their homes at substantial losses.

Dottie and Frank English moved from Pennsylvania to

the Midwest in 1993, but Dottie, in particular, remained actively involved in the issue as a board member of the EMR Alliance, an international network, and as a co-director of the Center for Public Information on EM Radiation.

Dottie English is confident that her concern and her activism are justified. Asked whether she overreacted to the issue, she responds firmly. "I *under*reacted, and I am sorry that we weren't better organized. I'm really sorry that I wasn't more vocal, more involved," English muses. Eventually, research will give us clear answers about EM field and EM radiation safety, she believes, but "it's going to take a lot of years. Until we get truly independent research, I don't think this issue is going to be solved," she says.

As Dottie English and hundreds of other people have learned, the research completed thus far is a mixed lot. There has never been a concerted, organized effort to understand whether EM fields and EM radiation are dangerous and, if so, how, despite the fact that EM fields and EM radiation are the by-products of electricity and increasingly common electrical devices such as cellular phones.

Our knowledge is based on a hodge-podge effort that nonetheless has produced compelling evidence that makes up in quantity at least some of what it lacks in quality. A handful of studies have found that children exposed to EM fields above a certain level—approximately 2 milligauss (a milligauss is the unit of measure for EM fields)—are approximately twice as likely to die from cancer as are children exposed to fewer than 2 milligauss. These studies are the most compelling and alarming of all the research, but they are not the only evidence that a problem exists. Adults exposed to EM fields and EM radiation on the job also are more likely to develop or die of cancer.

What really concerns scientists and public health specialists is that the levels associated with cancer are very low.

Indeed, millions of people experience 2 milligauss EM fields for extended periods every day. This research is inconclusive, however. What investigators have not yet found is an explanation for how EM fields and EM radiation at the very low levels we commonly encounter can cause cancer or any of the other health effects attributed to exposure. In other words, no one has yet found the mechanism of interaction—the smoking gun, so to speak.

That is not to say that research has not produced evidence pointing toward an explanation. Experimental results have produced at least four possible mechanisms. The hunt is on to prove or disprove whether exposure to EM fields or EM radiation causes cancer and other health problems. For scientists, this means that they must observe some or all of the following factors:

- *A strong statistical association.* If exposed people are only slightly more likely to develop cancer after exposure, that would be a weak association.
- *A consistent association.* The apparent link should be observable among people from diverse economic, racial, and geographic groups.
- *A specific association.* Exposure should produce a specific result—that is, a particular type of cancer.
- *A sequential association.* The exposure should precede the health effect.
- *A dose-response relationship.* As exposure conditions increase, the statistical association should grow stronger.
- *Scientific consistency.* There must be a plausible mechanism for the health effect, and the association should fit with prevailing scientific knowledge.
- *Agreement between human and animal studies.* Findings of cancer among humans should be reflected in findings of cancer among laboratory animals or animal cells or organs.

• *A scientific precedent.* There should be an analogous association between a causal agent and an effect.

EM fields and EM radiation are, based on all that we know now, unprecedented. No chemical or physical agent affects the human body in any of the ways that EM fields and EM radiation seem to.

As a result, scientists working to understand how EM fields and EM radiation might be dangerous are grappling with very complex problems on the cutting edge of research. The layers of difficult and unresolved questions overwhelm even some specialists. Stripping away the layers, however, reveals two basic questions: What effects occur? And how do they occur?

Scientists have tried to answer these questions through large-scale studies of people—known as epidemiological studies—and laboratory studies. This chapter summarizes some of the major findings. (In this relatively new and unexplored field, there are nonetheless more than 50 epidemiological studies and more than 12,000 laboratory studies. Appendix A details the major epidemiological findings on a study-by-study basis.) It spotlights the most widely recognized theories, questions, and effects, but it does not try to cover every facet.

If you read the original research, you will find that scientists have yet to determine whether it is more important to know the field strength, the wave shape, the frequency, the relationship of the field to the earth's geomagnetic field, the duration of exposure, or some other factor. You will also discover that every research result on EM fields and EM radiation health effects seems to raise more questions than it answers. For instance, researchers have observed changes at certain frequencies and power levels but not at others, with no obvious trends to explain the so-called windows.

It is important that you are aware of these issues, and it will help if you understand the research at at least a rudimentary level. Keep in mind, however, that there is uncertainty in all that we know—uncertainty that only more and better research can resolve. The scientific community, with few exceptions, accepts the need for a substantial research program that can answer at least some of the questions about EM fields and EM radiation—Why are research results uneven and inconsistent? What are the right studies to do? And in what order?

ELECTRICITY AND YOUR BODY

In fundamental ways, our bodies run on electricity. Electric signals help cells communicate, relay information to and from the brain, and keep our complex network of vital organs operating smoothly. Paradoxically, scientists on both sides of the debate believe this supports their views.

Scientists who believe that the research cannot be pieced together into a coherent picture to show an EM field and EM radiation risk (a small—and shrinking—but influential group) say that the laws of physics make health hazards impossible. They reason that low-level EM field and EM radiation signals are much weaker than the signals the body creates for normal cell functions, and that therefore the signals generated by an external field get lost in the body.

In contrast, a growing number of scientists have come to interpret the research as suggesting, but not proving, that EM field and radiation health effects are possible. Dr. David Savitz, a prominent researcher at the University of North Carolina, articulated this mainstream thinking in a 1993 article: "When the question is posed, Is there theoretical or empirical evidence that exposure to [EM] fields at commonly encountered levels poses a threat to health?, the answer must be a firm yes."

At EM radiation frequencies, scientists are starting to reach similar, though more tentative, conclusions. The late Dr. Cletus Kanavy, a scientist with the U.S. Air Force, argued shortly before his death in 1993 that, "A large amount of data exists, both animal experimental and human clinical evidence, to support the existence of chronic, nonthermal effects."

EM FIELDS AND EM RADIATION

EM fields and EM radiation are two types of electromagnetic energy. EM fields result from the flow of electric current—through a wire, for instance. The most common source of EM fields are power lines, such as the ones that carry electric current across the country and the ones that bring the current to your neighborhood or apartment building. In fact, any electric current produces an EM field (see Table 1).

EM radiation results from the acceleration of electrical charges, the building blocks of electricity. It comes from a diverse range of sources, such as radio and television broadcast antennas, cellular phones, and computer terminals (see Table 2).

Both EM fields and EM radiation are most readily understood as waves, similar to ocean waves and sound waves. The waves have characteristics such as frequency and wavelength that allow us to describe them and explain how they work.

EM fields have lower frequencies than EM radiation. Since frequency and wavelength are inversely related—one goes up as the other goes down—EM fields have shorter wavelengths than EM radiation. (Appendix B; "An EM Field and EM Radiation Primer," explains this in greater detail. See also the glossary that starts on page 227.)

Table 1

Common EM Field Sources

At Home

Electric power transmission lines

Electric power distribution lines

Appliances
   Air conditioners
   Blenders
   Clocks
   Electric blankets
   Electric mixers
   Electric razors
   Fluorescent lighting
   Hair dryers
   Heating pads
   Microwave ovens
   Portable electric heaters
   Power tools
   Refrigerators
   Televisions
   Toasters

Vacuum cleaners

In–home electric wiring and circuit boxes

At Work

Electric power transmission lines

Electric power distribution lines

Office equipment
   Calculators
   Fluorescent lighting
   Laser printers
   Pencil sharpeners
   Photocopiers
   Video display (computer) terminals

Office wiring
   Circuit boxes
   Transformers

Industrial equipment

Table 2

Common EM Radiation Sources

Baby monitors

Cellular phones

Cordless phones

Industrial equipment
   Radiofrequency sealers
   Medical systems

Local radio communications systems

Microwave ovens

Microwave phone links

Radar
   Police radar devices
   Military radar
   Weather radar

Radio broadcast signals

Satellite uplinks

Television broadcast signals

Video display (computer) terminals

Walkie–talkies

Wireless office networks

HEALTH RESEARCH

The health research on EM fields and EM radiation is inter-related but not interchangeable. EM radiation research comprises less study of human exposures and more study of animals than EM field research, in part because it is difficult to find a large group of people exposed in a uniform way to EM radiation.

EM radiation also is a much broader topic. The number of EM radiation frequencies is enormous, the number of forms EM radiation can take at each frequency is virtually limitless, and the thinking about where to target research is limited. As a result, we have more specific information about EM field exposures—most of which occur at one frequency, 60 hertz—than we do about EM radiation exposures that occur at millions of frequencies.

Nonthermal vs. Thermal Effects

By the start of World War II researchers knew that EM radiation could cause heating in the human body and that the heating could be harmful, even fatal. As a result, health research concentrated on determining how much heat individual body parts could absorb from EM radiation and yet return to normal temperature within a short period. Most of this research was done in the United States by the military, since EM radiation was just beginning to be widely used for radar and communications. By the end of the war, the military was the single largest user of EM radiation, a position it continues to hold.

Medical researchers were using EM radiation-generated heat on a limited basis for therapeutic purposes. Scientists rapidly learned to use higher and higher frequency EM radiation for military and medical applications.

Higher frequencies mean shorter wavelengths, which penetrate the body more readily, depositing more energy inside. More energy produces heat more rapidly. With the potential for faster and more efficient heating, scientists began assessing how efficiently the body and individual body parts could cool.

Sweat and the flow of blood are two ways the body reduces heat, and some body parts (such as the eyes) do not sweat and have limited blood flow, reducing their ability to cool. As a result, researchers hypothesized that EM radiation might produce cataracts, much as can other forms of electromagnetic energy such as ultraviolet light. In addition, they discovered from experiments involving people and from accidental exposures among radar operators and others that increasing EM radiation exposures caused discomfort leading to illness and, if not stopped in time, death. Clearly there was a limit to safe EM radiation heating.

After the war, a military team set the first EM radiation exposure standard, focusing exclusively on the heating problem. This approach established criteria that continue to influence thinking about EM radiation and EM fields today: if exposure does not produce significant heating, it must be safe. Indeed, the widely used voluntary industry guidelines for EM radiation exposures, known as the ANSI standard, addresses only thermal effects.

The military model dominated thinking into the late 1980s, but it no longer rules scientific thinking because researchers have demonstrated that nonthermal EM radiation and EM field exposures can cause changes in cell behavior, in the production of key hormones that regulate body functions, and in other physical processes.

EPIDEMIOLOGICAL STUDIES

Epidemiological studies are real to people because they are about real people. These studies involve large numbers of people, some of whom either were exposed to a suspected agent such as EM fields or EM radiation or who had developed or died of a disease thought to be linked to one or more agents. They use statistics to determine the probability that an agent is associated with an effect. Because they involve humans, their findings are directly useful in shaping personal and public responses to real or perceived hazards. Unfortunately, the complexity of our lives often makes it difficult for an epidemiological study to show a link that is not called into question by one or more variables. Indeed, epidemiological studies are not supposed to prove anything but merely to pinpoint trends.

For EM fields, epidemiological studies have been the driving force behind public concern. Because power lines are a primary source of EM fields, it is fairly easy for researchers to find a large group of people with common exposure conditions. To date, five studies have linked EM field exposures to childhood cancer, and thirty-nine have found associations between adult cancer and on-the-job exposure. A smaller number of studies have found a weak link between cancer among adults and EM field exposure at home.

EM radiation exposure is more difficult to study epidemiologically. EM radiation sources are not as uniform as power lines, and so it is relatively difficult to find a good study group. Only a couple of EM radiation studies have been completed for cancer. Their results suggest an association between EM radiation and cancer, but they raise too many questions about exposure conditions and other variables to provide unequivocal information. A slightly larger number of studies have suggested a link between EM radiation and reproductive problems.

EM Field Studies

The first, and most important, EM field study appeared in 1979. Dr. Nancy Wertheimer and Ed Leeper reported that children living near power distribution lines were roughly twice as likely to develop cancer as were other children.

Their study hypothesized that these power lines produced very weak magnetic fields that were a likely cause of the increased disease rate. Most scientists were skeptical of this theory. The Electric Power Research Institute (EPRI), a research association of electric utilities, offered a critical analysis that provided several alternative explanations for the cancer link. For instance, EPRI suggested that the power lines were taking the blame for harm caused by other (non–EM field) exposures such as air pollution from cars and trucks, since power distribution lines in the study area generally ran along streets.

Wertheimer and Leeper's results seemed highly implausible, so most observers expected Dr. David Savitz's attempt to replicate the study to disprove the findings. Commissioned by the New York State Power Lines Project, Savitz studied a similar group of children in Denver over a comparable period. His 1988 study confirmed Wertheimer and Leeper's findings, showing an association between power distribution lines and all types of childhood cancer, as well as between the lines and brain cancer in children.

At least three other studies of children in other areas and nations have confirmed Wertheimer and Leeper's conclusion. Another study using a different method of estimating exposure levels found no statistically significant increase due to exposure.

The childhood-cancer link to power frequency EM fields is generally considered the most convincing evidence that EM fields can be hazardous. Studies of adults living near power lines have produced less clear results. There are approximately an equal number of positive adult studies (those that find an association) as negative ones (those that don't). Adult cancer is more difficult to study because most adults have at some time in their lives been exposed to a wide range of chemicals and other agents known or suspected to cause cancer. Linking a single case of cancer to any one EM field or radiation exposure is very difficult.

To reduce the uncertainty, researchers have instead studied adults in their workplaces. Each workplace or occupation has many things in common, making it easier to look for cancer-causing factors. Seventeen occupational studies have linked EM field exposures to leukemia, five to brain cancer, four to male breast cancer, and thirteen to multiple types of cancer. Researchers have focused on jobs that involve extensive work on or near power lines and electronic equipment.

Certain types of cancer, including brain cancer and male breast cancer, stand out because they are rare compared to leukemia and other more common cancers. The breast cancer results made an unusually large impact on health researchers because male breast cancer and female breast cancer are similar diseases, and breast cancer is one of the leading causes of death in women in the United States. Only one study looking at breast cancer in women who worked with EM fields has been completed, and it found a link.

There are two reasons for caution in interpreting these occupational studies. First, workplaces are relatively dangerous areas that include a wide assortment of potential cancer-causing agents. Second, very few of the studies involved reliable measures of worker exposures. The most common way of "measuring" exposure was to assume that a worker was exposed if he or she worked in an "electrical occupation." Attempts in the early to mid-1990s to have workers wear meters to measure EM field exposures on an ongoing basis may prove useful, but the meaning of the measurements remains unclear.

Determining exposure conditions with precision is a major uncertainty in all of the human studies. Human exposures depend on variables that are difficult to account for in a large-scale study. For example, should scientists be concerned primarily with the duration of exposure? The duration of exposure above a certain level? The source of the exposure (e.g., an alarm clock vs. a computer terminal)? Or is it even more complicated, dependent on the amount of electricity being used by your neighbors (thereby drawing more current past your house)? Meters that are worn or that are located throughout a home or workplace may not be able to account for key variables.

Wertheimer and Leeper developed a method of wire coding for power distribution lines that may be a clever method of averaging long-term exposures in homes, or it may be a false measure altogether. Many of the human studies have found cancer links with estimated exposures based on wire coding but failed to find links using short-term measurements.

The Wertheimer-Leeper coding system grouped houses as either high-current or low-current according to the type of power distribution wires nearby. (See Chapter 2 for a more detailed explanation.) They confirmed the accuracy of the groupings by taking a series of sample measurements. Several subsequent research teams have confirmed that the coding system is reliable. What is not known is whether it accurately accounts for the right variable or set of variables.

EM Radiation Studies

Studies of people exposed to EM radiation are rare but suggestive. A Polish research team found in a series of analyses that Polish military personnel exposed to EM radiation at higher levels and for longer periods than other military personnel were more likely to die from cancer, including some types of leukemia. More recently, a Croation team found that workers exposed to EM radiation experienced chromosomal changes consistent with the development of cancer, and observed similar chromosomal changes in human and animal cells exposed in laboratories.

Investigations of cancer clusters—significantly elevated cancer rates within a community—have identified EM radiation as a possible cause, but this method of investigation rarely draws firm links. For example, the state of Hawaii investigated fourteen cases of childhood leukemia near a Navy EM radiation transmitter on Oahu and found a "weak association" between the disease and the children's proximity to the device, but could go no further.

The EM radiation issue will not be resolved without more and better epidemiological studies. Laboratory research involving animals, cells, and animal organs presents relatively strong evidence of a link between EM radiation and cancer.

THE HUNT FOR MECHANISMS

The epidemiological evidence cannot stand alone. Scientists have done more than 12,000 experiments involving animals, cells, and animal organs and either EM fields or EM radiation in an effort to understand and explain how exposure conditions that do not produce heating might cause harm. Identifying nonthermal effects does not explain them. The single biggest research question remains: What is the mechanism of interaction?

At least four theories are considered plausible, but even their proponents concede that they are either many small steps or one giant leap from solving the mechanism puzzle. If EM fields and EM radiation are one day linked conclusively to health hazards, the odds are good that there will be multiple mechanisms.

Cell Interaction

The cell is the primary unit of all living organisms, comprising a mass of protein that is subdivided into two parts—the cytoplasm and the nucleus. The nucleus contains DNA, the genetic basis of life. The cytoplasm envelops the nucleus and other components of the cell.

All animal cells, including human cells, are bordered by cell membranes. These membranes are semipermeable, and they regulate the flow of vital electrical signals in and out of the cell. The roles of these signals are to control cell reproduction, muscle contraction, and other critical activities. Upsetting the signals can have an effect on the cell.

The most thoroughly studied aspect of cell function is the effect EM fields have on the flow of calcium ions in and out of the cell. These ions, or charged particles, play a central role in relaying information vital to cell functions. As early as the mid-1970s, researchers found that EM fields near power frequencies and at EM radiation frequencies could change the rate at which calcium flowed out of the cell. Subsequent research also showed an effect on the rate at which calcium entered the cell.

What perplexed the researchers, and continues to vex them, is that the effects occurred at some frequencies but not at others. Early research, done using chicken brains, by

Dr. Suzanne Bawin and Dr. Ross Adey found that calcium flow out of the cell decreased when the cell was exposed to EM fields at 6 hertz and 16 hertz, but not at other frequencies. In addition, at these frequencies the effects occurred only with certain power levels. Adey has since honed this finding and believes that the flow of signal carriers into and out of the cell—known as cell communication—constitutes a plausible mechanism to explain how EM fields can be linked to cancer development.

Dr. Carl Blackman of the Environmental Protection Agency found that he could *increase* the flow of calcium out of the cells with some frequencies in the power frequency range but not with others. He also found that certain power levels produced effects while others did not. Though he used different frequencies and power levels from Bawin and Adey, he confirmed their report of "windows"—small openings where effects were seen.

Blackman later took the research a step further. He discovered that a static magnetic field—that is, a magnetic field that is not changing direction at any frequency—could alter the cell's response. He could, in effect, open new windows by applying a static magnetic field.

Finally, Blackman also showed in more recent research that not only calcium ions but also other molecules are affected by EM fields. The windows effect suggests that EM field effects are nonlinear—that is, there is no dose-response relationship between exposure and effect.

Other researchers have tried to observe the effects of changes in calcium flow out of brain cells using whole animals in their studies. These investigations used surrogates for calcium flow by looking at biological changes linked to calcium flow. None of the studies found effects similar to those observed using animal cells or organs alone, but the researchers readily acknowledged that their use of surrogates was an untested and potentially unreliable method.

Cyclotron Resonance

Dr. Abe Liboff of Oakland University in Rochester, Michigan, has hypothesized that a phenomenon known as cyclotron resonance may explain EM field and EM radiation interactions at the cell-membrane level. He theorized that ions (e.g., calcium ions) cross the cell membrane along helical structures. Helixes are rotating down or up ramps—sort of like the ramps you use to drive in or out of a large parking garage. As the ion moves along the helix, it has a frequency and will absorb energy at that frequency, known as the cyclotron resonance frequency. This absorption, presumably involving EM fields or, more likely, EM radiation, affects how the ion behaves when it crosses the cell membrane. If the energy disrupts the ion's behavior, it might lead to health effects.

Melatonin, Circadian Rhythms, and Cancer

At the base of the brain is the pineal gland, which produces a hormone called melatonin. The pineal gland regulates day and night for us—circadian rhythms—and helps animals navigate. In the early 1980s, scientists began studying the effect EM fields had on pineal glands in animals. They found that exposed animals sometimes grew disoriented and often lost track of day and night. They also noted that exposures reduced production of melatonin.

When other researchers studied the effect of EM fields on human melatonin levels, they found similar results, particularly the influence on our ability to regulate day and night. The suppression of melatonin levels owing to EM field exposures raises several possible concerns, since pineal function is linked to a wide range of illnesses and diseases. In fact, two melatonin-related effects reflect current concerns about EM field exposures—cancer and depression.

One of the things that melatonin does is slow the growth of cancerous cells in laboratory animals. Reduced melatonin levels are associated with increased breast cancer rates in rats, for example. As a result, the hypothesis that reduced melatonin levels due to EM field exposures are linked to the cancer findings seems to hold promise.

Disrupted circadian rhythms are associated in research with psychological disturbances such as depression and emotional disorders. For instance, lower than normal melatonin levels are linked to seasonal affective disorder (SAD), which occurs during winter months apparently as a result of light deprivation. Depression associated with SAD often is treated with scheduled light exposures to increase melatonin levels.

Magnetite

Another possible mechanism is the presence of magnetite in the brain. Found in humans for the first time in the early 1990s, magnetite is a magnetic material commonly found in other materials. A special panel reviewing EM field health effects for the Department of Energy in 1992 and 1993 reported that "the recent discovery of magnetite in the human brain could change the picture in a very significant way. The magnetic properties of this material . . . provide a physically plausible mechanism by which magnetic fields might perturb biological systems."

The mechanism of magnetite interaction is pure conjecture, but the significance for EM fields and EM radiation may be great. As the Energy Department panel concluded, "The essential point to take away from all of this work is that a cellular-level coupling of magnetic fields to biological systems is physically plausible and does not violate any physical principles."

As research results accumulated and led researchers to these theories, most scientists stopped asking whether nonthermal exposures could cause changes and began asking whether these changes are harmful. The body is resilient, and it will withstand some changes. It was no longer a question of, Are there nonthermal effects? Instead, the question became, Are nonthermal effects harmful?

None of the proposed mechanisms has yet gained broad scientific acceptance as proof of an EM field or EM radiation link to cancer. There is as yet no proof that a mechanism exists—a smoking gun—linking nonthermal exposures to human harm.

SPECIFIC EFFECTS

The way researchers hunt for mechanisms is to study animals, animal organs, and human and animal cells under controlled EM field and EM radiation exposure conditions. They want to observe a mechanism at work causing or producing a specific health condition. Here, then, are some of the effects that laboratory investigators are concentrating on and their importance to human health.

Tumor Growth and Cancer Promotion

Neither EM fields nor EM radiation *cause* cancer per se, most researchers agree. What they may do is *promote* cancer. Cancer is a multistage process that requires an "initiator" that makes a cell or group of cells abnormal. Everyone has cancerous cells in his or her body. Cancer—the disease as we think of it—occurs when these cancerous cells grow uncontrollably.

Researchers have found that cancerous cells grow and reproduce more rapidly when they are exposed to EM fields or EM radiation than when they are not exposed. A two-part experiment provides interesting evidence of this.

In one part of the experiment, Drs. Jack McLean and Maria Stuchly, both with the Canadian government, put a known tumor-promoting chemical on the skin of mice before exposing some of the mice to power frequency EM fields. The exposed mice developed more than three times as many tumors as the nonexposed mice.

The complementary experiment by the same research team used the same tumor promoter with cancer cells. The exposed cells had double the number of cancer cells as the nonexposed controls. Earlier research had identified a similar cancer promotion effect for EM radiation.

Another important study, by Dr. Stephen Cleary and his colleagues at Virginia Commonwealth University, found that brain tumor cells exposed to EM radiation reproduced at an accelerated rate for as long as five days after exposure. They also found a window effect, much like Adey's discovery at lower frequencies, whereby effects occurred only under specific exposure conditions. When the exposure level increased, the cell growth decreased.

The fact that the effect lingered raised the possibility that cumulative exposures could have a multiple effect. For people who move in and out of EM radiation, this might raise concerns. In addition, because the experiments were done at frequencies near to those used by cellular telephones, the findings later became central to the debate over the role cellular phone emissions might play in brain cancer.

Perhaps the most significant and one of the most controversial studies found that rats exposed to microwave frequency EM radiation developed cancer at a significantly higher rate than unexposed rats. The study is the largest and most thorough of several such investigations, and one of the nation's most respected researchers, Dr. Arthur Guy, formerly of the University of Washington, led the study.

Genetics

EM fields and EM radiation seem to affect the way the body's basic building blocks reproduce—a process called RNA transcription.

Dr. Reba Goodman of Columbia University and Dr. Ann Henderson of Hunter College, both in New York City, have shown in their pioneering work that RNA transcription is affected by EM fields. They also have found that different frequency exposures seem to produce different effects, possibly helping to explain the windows phenomenon. While the meaning of this finding remains uncertain, it suggests that some health effects could begin at this very basic level.

Behavior

Though studied only sporadically, the EM field–depression link resonates in the research. As recently as 1992, investigators documented a doubling of symptoms of depression among people living along power line rights-of-way, the land on both sides of electric power transmission lines. This finding echoes the theories that surrounded the microwave EM radiation exposure of the United States Embassy in Moscow by the Soviet Union in the 1960s. When the beaming was discovered, U.S. officials believed that the Soviets were trying to influence the emotional states of American workers.

Another behavioral effect identified but never researched thoroughly is the finding by Dr. Kurt Salzinger of Polytechnic University in Brooklyn, New York, that exposure to power frequency EM fields can significantly retard learning in rats. Salzinger exposed rat fetuses during gestation and for their first eight days of life. At ninety days, the rats were trained to perform a set of tasks.

Exposed rats had response rates as much as 20 percent slower than nonexposed rates. Coming almost three months after exposure, the findings suggested that learning can be slowed long after exposure.

A military pilot accidentally exposed to EM radiation for five minutes may have provided evidence that this delayed effect occurs in humans as well. Following the inadvertent exposure, the pilot experienced partial loss of his short-term memory. Gradually, his memory returned.

Reproduction

Fetuses in animals and humans are susceptible to harm, and so researchers have focused on the possible effects of EM fields and EM radiation on the reproductive process. One of the most important studies was done in the early 1980s in Spain by Drs. José Delgado and Jocelyn Leal.

Delgado and Leal exposed chicken embryos (eggs) to both EM fields and EM radiation and found a "consistent and powerful" effect: fetal malformations. Key to the experiments was the pulsed wave shape of the exposure signals. Pulsed emissions reach their peak levels very quickly—for example, in a millionth of a second—and as a result cause biological changes in ways different from emissions that rise to peak levels gradually.

By coincidence, the EM radiation from computer monitors (VDTs, or video display terminals) has wave shapes similar to those Delgado used. This spurred concerns about VDT effects on pregnancy. Indeed, the Delgado-Leal experiment is largely responsible for the spate of epidemiological studies of VDT reproductive effects during the 1980s and early 1990s.

Researchers in Sweden picked up on the coincidence and exposed mice fetuses *in utero* to simulated VDT EM radiation emissions and found a pattern of malformations and miscarriages.

The Delgado study also led to an international project to test the findings, called the Henhouse Project. In that set of experiments, researchers in four nations independently tried to do the same experiment using identical equipment, laboratory setups, and eggs. Overall, the project confirmed the Delgado results, though some labs produced positive findings while others were negative.

Vision

Because EM radiation at thermal levels is known to cause cataracts, researchers have an ongoing interest in assessing whether nonthermal levels might also produce cataracts. The results are inconclusive and controversial.

Researchers also are evaluating the effect of EM radiation on key eye components. Henry Kues of the Johns Hopkins University Applied Physics Laboratory, perhaps the premier researcher in this area, has found evidence that exposure can harm both the cones and the rods that help us see. Cones provide color discrimination and visual acuity, while rods are photoreceptors that help provide night vision. Kues found that both cones and rods failed after exposure, and then regained their capacities at differing rates. The rods recovered to a great extent within a week, but the cones suffered long-term damage.

THE RESEARCH GAP

The data are inconclusive and will remain unsettled probably for at least another decade. There is too much evidence of health effects to dismiss scientific and public concern, and there are too many unresolved questions to identify with confidence clear, unquestioned risks.

We are witnessing the impact of the research lag of the early to mid-1980s, when the federal government ignored the advice of its experts and reduced its small but ambitious research program to a shell (see Chapter 7). Other nations—in particular, Sweden—took the international lead. Now Americans are playing catch-up, while people concerned about what they have heard and what they know search for guidance and leadership. Sweden, drawing on its aggressive research efforts and placing credence in the conclusions its scientists have reached, is developing health-based rules to protect children living near power lines.

Your Exposures and What You Can Do

CHAPTER 2

YOUR EM FIELD
EXPOSURES

Y OU ARE EXPOSED TO EM FIELDS VIRTUALLY EVERY MINUTE OF
every day. That should reassure you. If all EM field exposures caused cancer, cancer would be as common as electricity. The chances are relatively small that you will develop
cancer or other ailments as a result of EM field exposures,
even if EM fields can be harmful.

This does not mean that you should ignore the EM fields
risk, however. Statistics mask the fact that some people may
be at greater risk than others, so the first challenge you face
is to evaluate whether you might be in a high-risk group.
Children, teachers, and other staff members in schools located near transmission lines may be a vulnerable group, for
example, as may be people working with electric current all
the time, such as phone company technicians or people constantly exposed at close range, as are some electric-blanket
users. Less obviously, people whose homes are wired incor-
rectly or are improperly grounded face potential hazards.

In short, one of the biggest challenges in determining possible EM field risks is accurately assessing whether you, your family, or your co-workers are experiencing unusually high exposures.

This chapter explains how and where you are exposed to EM fields. It will help you put your EM field exposures into perspective—when exposures are likely to be significant and when they are not—and also help you think through some of the decisions you can make. In Chapter 3 you will find practical tips for reducing your exposures from a comprehensive list of EM field sources, including computers and other office devices, home and office wiring, home appliances, and factory equipment.

The EMF Book assumes that you want to know how to reduce your EM field exposures regardless of the sources. This may mean you will need to make changes in your home and office. It certainly means that you must make a comprehensive survey of your home; your workplace; the schools your children attend if you have children; and any other place where you or your family spend a lot of time. You will find that identifying EM field sources is not difficult in most instances, once you know what you are looking for.

THEY ARE EVERYWHERE

The first thing you should know about EM fields and EM radiation is that they are everywhere. In an average day you probably are exposed to EM fields from dozens of sources—your bedside clock, your hair dryer, your electric toothbrush, your electric oven, your microwave oven, the wiring inside your house, the wires that run outside your house. You get the picture. If it runs on electricity or if it carries electricity, it generates an EM field.

Where Does Electricity Come From?

Power plants generate electrical charges for transmission and distribution to consumers. These electrical charges make up the electricity that powers our world. At the plant the charges are pumped onto transmission lines. The amount of charge that is put on the line is the voltage, as in "high-voltage" line. The common voltages for high-voltage transmission lines in the United States are 69,000 volts (69 kilovolts), 115 kilovolts, 230 kilovolts, 500 kilovolts, and 765 kilovolts. Transmission lines are the thick cables you often see running along tall metal towers. Often these are called high-tension lines.

Transmission lines eventually drop off some of the voltage for local distribution. Each drop-off point requires a sub-station, which is a complex network of devices that reduce—or "transform"—the voltage sharply, usually to a level between 5 kilovolts and 35 kilovolts. These are primary distribution voltages, and primary distribution lines carry electricity to secondary distribution lines that, in turn, drop off the electricity directly to consumers.

Distribution lines are most often strung on telephone poles, though in many communities built during the past decade they are buried underground. Many telephone poles carry lines for multiple purposes—phones, cable television, and electricity. You can identify power distribution lines because they rest at each pole on insulators that look a little like ceramic mushrooms. You may see more than one set of lines on a single set of telephone poles, probably indicating that the route includes both a primary distribution line and a secondary distribution line.

The secondary distribution lines carry 115 volt and 230 volt current. The voltage is converted from the primary to the secondary lines by a transformer, which serves much the same function as a substation but on a smaller scale. At 120 volts, the electric current can be delivered to homes, most of which operate at this voltage. Large energy users such as factories and large office buildings receive 240 volt current.

Inside a home or business, the electricity is distributed by internal wiring after passing through a circuit breaker or, in older homes, a fuse box. These devices ensure that the internal wiring is protected against a sudden pulse or burst of electricity coming into the home, such as might occur if lightning hit a local power line. Aside from producing a pulse of EM field, an electrical surge can quickly ruin delicate electric circuits in appliances and computers, and can even cause fires. The circuit breaker is vitally important from an EM field perspective as well, since it is where an electrician can most readily balance the flow of current into and out of your home.

Most residences use single-phase wiring. This means that only one of the three wires connecting all the appliances and devices (switches, lamps, appliances, etc.) is carrying current. Electricians say it is the "hot" wire. A second wire is the return wire, carrying current back to the electrical grid. The third wire is the ground wire.

Most transmission and distribution systems use three-phase wiring, in which three wires are hot but their wave cycles are carefully offset into three steps. Imagine the wave cycle divided into thirds; at any given moment, one wire's wave is in the first third of the cycle, the second wire's wave is in the middle cycle, and the third wire's wave is in the third cycle.

All electrical systems must be grounded for safety. The ground wire, or connection, ensures that any excess or unintended current in the system is allowed to flow into the earth so that it can return to the transmission and distribution network. All alternating current, which is what the electric power system is, needs a complete circuit. If, for example, a frayed hot wire comes in contact with the frame of an electric stove, the metal frame of the stove will be electrified. If you touched it, you would provide a route for the current to "return to ground," and you would receive a strong, potentially fatal, shock.

Proper grounding is done at the point where the distribution system enters your home or workplace—the drop-off point or point of entry. Ideally, a ground wire is run from the electric meter or the circuit breaker box directly into the ground, giving electricity an easy route back to the distribution system, which also is grounded. Each major appliance and all outlets in a home circuit should be grounded as well.

All too often the ground wire is not run directly to the earth but instead connects to metal plumbing pipes that eventually come into contact with the earth. As a result, the pipes carry currents, sometimes high currents, and produce EM fields. Often, these currents on the plumbing are a primary source of EM fields. This and other improper grounding methods also tend to unbalance a home's circuit, generating substantial field levels. In and around many homes, plumbing-based grounding that disrupts the current balance and phasing is the major source of EM fields.

POWER LINE EXPOSURES

About 20 million Americans are regularly exposed to EM fields from power lines at levels higher than 2 milligauss (the common unit of measurement for EM fields), which some experts believe is the threshold for safety. In a small number of instances, people living very near substations and transmission lines may be experiencing fields significantly higher than 2 milligauss. In cities such as Philadelphia, where row houses predominate in many neighborhoods, utilities string distribution lines by attaching the wires directly to the houses rather than on telephone poles running through alleys or across yards. Fields inside homes near these lines can be unusually high.

Most people are regularly exposed to just 1 milligauss or less, even though they may periodically experience maximum levels greater than 10 milligauss. The number of people exposed to an excess of 2 milligauss from internal wiring (the electrical circuit inside your home or workplace) and appliance use is unknown, since investigators have found substantial variation in homes.

There is nothing magical—or conclusive—about the 2 milligauss threshold. Higher levels may not be more hazardous than lower levels, though most experts consider it common sense to assume that they are. At the same time, 1 milligauss and 1.5 milligauss fields may not be safer than 3 milligauss ones.

Public concern has focused on power lines more than on appliances because exposure to power line EM fields is involuntary and usually occurs for long periods. You can dry your hair with a towel instead of an electric hair dryer if you are concerned, and you can limit the amount of time you use the hair dryer. But the power distribution lines that run through your suburban neighborhood or your urban highrise apartment are permanent, and electric current runs through them constantly.

Occasionally, you will hear that electric razors, electric hair dryers, and other common home appliances appear to be more dangerous than transmission and distribution lines because they emit higher field levels. This is misleading. It is highly unlikely that brief exposures, even at the relatively high levels that some appliances produce, are more likely to pose a hazard than lower exposures that last for eight hours or more. EM fields do not seem to act like X rays and other types of ionizing radiation, which can harm you at high intensities no matter how brief your exposure.

Appliances and Other Common Exposures

Many surveys have measured emissions levels around appliances and electrical devices. The U.S. Environmental Protection Agency (EPA) has summarized some of the findings. A snapshot of the EPA's data appears in Table 3.

The numbers show that within one foot of many appliances, EM field levels are high. At two feet, far fewer produce exposures greater than 2 milligauss, and at four feet the EM fields from most appliances can not be distinguished from background levels.

The EPA excluded electric blankets, which produce high EM field levels to which many people are exposed for long periods while they sleep. Tests have shown EM fields of more than 200 milligauss within six inches of an electric blanket. New, reduced-emission electric blankets produce fields of less than 20 milligauss at the same distance.

HOW TO THINK ABOUT YOUR EXPOSURES

You have to decide whether and to what extent you want to protect yourself and your family, based on the incomplete and sometimes contradictory evidence linking EM fields to cancer, learning disorders, and other harmful effects. Complicating the issue is the uncertainty about what aspects of EM fields, if any, are hazardous. Is it the strength of the field? In that case you must lower your exposure levels. Or is it some other, less obvious factor (such as your orientation to the earth's geomagnetic field while you are exposed to

---

Table 3

EM Field Emission Levels in Milligauss from Appliances and Electrical Devices

Source	6 inches	1 foot	2 feet	4 feet
AIR CLEANERS	180	35	5	1
BABY MONITORS	6	1	*	*
BATTERY CHARGERS	30	3	*	*
BLACK & WHITE TV	–	3	*	*
BLENDERS	70	10	2	*
CAN OPENERS	600	150	20	2
CEILING FANS	–	3	*	*
CLOTHES DRYER	3	2	*	*
COFFEEMAKERS	7	*	*	*
COLOR TV	–	7	2	*
COPY MACHINES	90	20	7	1
CROCKPOTS	6	1	*	*
DIAL CLOCKS	–	15	2	*
DIGITAL CLOCKS	–	1	*	*
DISHWASHERS	20	10	4	*
ELECTRIC DRILLS	150	30	4	*
ELECTRIC OVENS	9	4	*	*
PENCIL SHARPENERS	200	70	20	2
ELECTRIC RANGES	30	8	2	*
FAX MACHINES	6	*	*	*
FLUORESCENT LIGHTS	40	6	2	*
FOOD PROCESSORS	30	6	2	*
GARBAGE DISPOSALS	80	10	2	*
IRONS	8	1	*	*
MICROWAVE OVENS	200	40	10	2
MIXERS	100	10	1	*
PORTABLE HEATERS	100	20	4	*
POWER SAWS	200	40	5	*
REFRIGERATORS	2	2	1	*
STEREO EQUIPMENT	1	*	*	*
TOASTERS	10	3	*	*
VACUUM CLEANERS	300	60	10	1
VDTs (Color Monitor)	14	5	2	*
WASHING MACHINES	20	7	1	*

– = No readings taken or no data available.
* = Readings taken, EM field indistinguishable from ambient.
Note: All measurements are median values obtained while each appliance was operating under normal circumstances.

a man-made source)? That presents a different, far more complex problem.

The uncertainty need not discourage you from taking precautions. Many scientists have concluded that in the absence of clear evidence it makes sense to assume that you want to be exposed for the shortest possible time and to the lowest possible field levels.

On this premise, in 1989 a team of researchers at Carnegie Mellon University in Pittsburgh, Pennsylvania, popularized the phrase "prudent avoidance" to describe a strategy of reducing exposures by no-cost or low-cost methods that cause minimal disruptions. Under this approach, moving a crib away from the side of a room where EM fields are high is "prudent" because distance is one way to lower exposure levels; moving out of the house probably is not. Other scientists and policy makers have refined and adapted this idea, and it remains the most widely accepted guidance on EM field exposure.

Prudent avoidance is based on the concept of cost-benefit analysis, which assumes that you can determine what is a reasonable amount to spend to reduce or eliminate a risk. Prudent avoidance can be a useful method for comparing one type of risk to another—EM fields to toxic chemicals, for instance. For individuals, its major limit is that it assumes you can and will put a price tag on your health or the health of your loved ones—something that many people find distasteful, difficult, or both.

Unless and until researchers prove EM fields either hazardous or safe beyond reasonable doubt, what is prudent for one person may be unacceptable to another. For instance, the cancer risk may convince you to spend hundreds of dollars to correct wiring conditions in your home. Or you might be willing only to turn off your computer monitor when you are not working at it. Of course, you may decide to do nothing. The choices you make will be influenced by a variety of factors in your life, such as what you can afford, whether you have the option of turning off your computer monitor and other work-control issues, and where your kids go to school.

Reducing exposures makes sense, even though no one can guarantee that it will make you, your family, or your co-workers safer. Most of the time, simple steps will significantly reduce the amount and time of your exposures. By learning what you *can* do, you will gain the ability to search out EM field sources in a room, an office, a factory, and a home. As with most known and possible environmental hazards, awareness and understanding are the single most important step toward personal protection.

You also should know that electric power utilities, employers, landlords, and electrical equipment manufacturers have economic and legal motivations to reduce exposures. Keith Florig, a researcher with Resources for the Future in Washington, D.C., has identified several such motivations. Reducing liability risks and lowering the potential expense of retrofitting equipment are significant incentives that may help drive the movement to reduce exposures in the absence of indisputable evidence that a risk exists.

THE MAIN EXPOSURE VARIABLES

There are three primary variables about EM fields you should understand and apply: field strength, distance from field sources, and duration of exposure.

Reducing *field strength* is something engineers and product designers can do most effectively and usually at the least cost before an electrical product is manufactured. A Swedish scientist has concluded that the cost of reducing EM field emissions from computer terminals is about $1 per unit during mass production, compared to approximately $100 to retrofit each unit after it is in use. Many manufacturers are heeding this finding, and the number of appliances and devices using EM field–reducing designs is increasing steadily. When public concern arose about EM fields from electric blankets, for example, manufacturers quickly redesigned the blanket wiring and introduced reduced-emission models. In addition, engineers have found a multitude of ways to arrange power transmission and distribution lines to lower field levels.

For the purpose of minimizing EM fields from electrical wires, there are two key concerns: balance and phasing. A common household circuit is balanced if the amount of current entering a house is equal to the amount leaving the house. Electricians seek to balance current, but a balanced circuit is almost impossible to sustain. In addition, common but ill-advised wiring shortcuts usually unbalance household circuits. Just as electricians try to balance current load in homes, your electric utility tries to balance the current load on the distribution network comprising several homes.

The second key is phasing. EM fields, by definition, affect one another. When two EM fields of equal strength meet while one is at its peak strength and the other is at its lowest strength, they will cancel each other out. This concept is sometimes known as *countervailing fields*, and it occurs when fields are "in phase." It also requires the sources of the fields—the conducting wires—to be a uniform distance apart. When fields are out of phase, they produce net fields that can range from very weak to very strong; just as fields can subtract from one another, they can add to one another.

Transmission, distribution, and internal wiring systems can be designed to always be in phase and to always balance, but in practice this is rarely the case. All it takes is one tree branch to move a line out of phase. In your home, a wiring shortcut can wreak havoc with the balance and phasing of your system. In addition, improper but common wiring for multiple-switch circuits (such as a lamp you can turn on with switches at opposite ends of a room) will produce strong EM fields in a room. Finally, while modern electrical systems use a type of wire cable that has all three wires wrapped together, inadvertently but effectively reducing EM fields through phasing, old homes (generally forty or more years old) may still have wiring systems that produce consistently high fields because the wires are far apart and out of phase.

You can reduce field strength. Some devices can be rewired or retrofitted to reduce emissions, though this is a more expensive option that requires a specialist. In addition, special metal alloys can reduce field levels effectively but usually at considerable cost. The challenge of finding inexpensive and practical solutions is spurring scientists to develop creative, low-cost ways of reducing EM field emissions. For instance, a researcher at the Stevens Institute of Technology in Hoboken, New Jersey, has developed a type of netting that he says will significantly reduce emissions when it is stretched under power lines like a circus safety net or used like a fence around power substations and transformers. Another innovator at Catholic University in Washington, D.C., has devised an electronic method that one computer equipment maker is using to nullify computer EM fields. Another company produces a large metal band that wraps around computer monitors to mitigate the emissions.

Once you learn to identify emissions sources, you can use your knowledge to reduce your exposure. By learning the differences among power line configurations, you can avoid areas where you suspect or know the field levels are high.

When you buy a computer terminal, choose one that meets Sweden's low-emissions guidelines (see Chapter 3 for more information). Most new terminals meet these guidelines.

Increasing the *distance* between you and the field source is one of the least expensive and useful things you can do. EM fields lose their energy very quickly as they travel: At two feet from a source, the field strength is one-fourth to one-eighth what it is at one foot. Some electric bedside clocks emit surprisingly strong EM fields, for example, and you will reduce your exposure while you sleep by moving the clock farther from your bed. If your favorite chair backs up to a wall that contains the electric circuit box for your house, move the chair. Consider rearranging your office so that your desk is as far away as possible from electrical devices such as copiers, and computers.

You should spend as little time as possible in an EM field. If the fields are produced by distribution lines outside your home, you and your family will be unavoidably exposed while you are home, which for most people is at least eight hours daily. On the other hand, you may be able to arrange your office so that the laser printer is across the room and your desk is the farthest possible distance from electric cables that run inside one of the walls of your office.

One other factor you need to consider is EM field pulses, or spikes, which occur commonly when electrical devices turn on or off, or when they rapidly increase or decrease the amount of energy they are using. For example, each time a photocopier starts to copy it requires a surge of electricity, producing a short EM field pulse. A device in your computer called a flyback transformer emits EM field pulses about seventy times per second. Telephone repairmen who work with older equipment are exposed to pulses every time an electromechanical switch is thrown, which is what happens each time someone makes a phone call. These pulses may be important in determining health effects, as explained in Chapter 1. Most of the time, pulses are predictable if you know how a given device works, and you may be able to get information from manufacturers that can help you figure this out. Unfortunately, there is no way of "seeing" pulses without a high-quality EM field measuring device (a gauss meter).

MEASUREMENTS

Accurately measuring EM fields is difficult. Simple, inexpensive gauss meters starting at less than $100 are easy to use but may provide imprecise readings. Sophisticated meters offer accurate and useful information, but only if you are properly trained in how to use them and how to interpret the data they produce. Currently there are several dozen gauss meters offered to consumers. (You can obtain a list by sending one dollar and a stamped, self-addressed envelope to Microwave News, P.O. Box 1799, Grand Central Station, New York, NY 10163.)

In 1992, the Environmental Protection Agency released the results of laboratory tests it had conducted on thirty gauss meters. The accuracy of the devices varied widely, with some showing errors of more than 100 percent in reading field levels under carefully controlled laboratory conditions. Most had error ranges of less than 20 percent, but the data raise doubts about your ability to get precise readings using many gauss meters.

A reputable engineer will tell you directly that there is a degree of uncertainty in his readings. If you take measurements yourself, be aware that your readings are likely no more than rough estimates of exposure levels. Still, these data are helpful so long as you do not get hung up on a 2 milligauss threshold. You should be interested primarily in two questions:

• *First, what range do the readings fall into—0.01–1 milligauss, 1–10 milligauss, 10–100 milligauss, or more than 100 milligauss?* For practical purposes, each order of magnitude difference is more important than are distinctions between 1 milligauss and 3 milligauss or between 13 milligauss and 20 milligauss. If the readings are between 0.01 and 1 milligauss, you are least likely to be at risk. This level is common. If the readings are between 1 and 10 milligauss, you will have to judge whether to take precautions, depending on the reliability of the measurement, the source of the EM field, and the duration of the exposure. You should repeat the measurement at other times and on other days to see how the field varies under different conditions.

If the readings are 10–100 milligauss or greater than 100 milligauss, you definitely should repeat the measurements at other times and on other days. Identify EM field sources (see Chapter 3) and consider methods for reducing exposures. Exposures of 10–100 milligauss are uncommon and exposures of 100 milligauss or greater are rare.

• *Second, are there significant variations within your home (or office)?* If you find very high levels on the side nearest a power distribution line but much lower levels on the opposite end of the house, not only will you be able to come up with a possible explanation for the source of the fields but you also can respond. In addition, you might notice "hot spots"—localized areas where field levels rise sharply. If you want to find a likely hot spot or just double check that your gauss meter is working, take a reading near an electric fan or an electric dial-face alarm clock (digital clocks emit much lower levels). You should see some high numbers.

If you decide to test your home, office, or factory for EM

fields—whether you hire a consultant, request a utility survey, or do it yourself—proceed with a clear plan. The plan should include the locations you want to measure and the number of measurements you want to take at each location. Take readings at the center of each room, near outside walls, and in the vicinity of electrical appliances, particularly if you suspect the device contributes significantly to field levels. Make detailed notes about conditions while you take readings: the time of day, the number of electrical devices in use at your home or workplace, the likely EM field sources (whether visible or hidden), and other observations. Remember that EM fields travel through walls unimpeded, so be alert to potential hazards that might not be apparent. Before you begin, you might draw a floor plan on which you can indicate EM field sources.

One of the biggest difficulties researchers have had interpreting scientific studies is the discrepancy among measurement conditions in different studies. For instance, readings of EM fields from power lines at 11:00 A.M. on a fall morning will almost always show lower field levels than would readings at the same location at 2:00 P.M. on a hot summer afternoon, when everyone in the neighborhood is running an air conditioner, or at 7:00 P.M. on weeknights, when most people have their TVs on. EM field strength is directly related to the amount of current flowing, and the current flow increases with each additional air conditioner, TV, or other appliance.

Hundreds of EM field measurements in homes and offices have produced a frustrating, murky picture of exposure levels. Fields are produced externally by transmission lines and distribution lines; internally by home or workplace wiring systems, as well as by currents induced by what is known as ground currents (excess electric current returning to the power distribution system though the earth); and locally by virtually every electrical appliance and device. All of these sources must be accounted for in assessing your exposure.

Researchers have used a variety of measurement methods with varying degrees of success. These include taking readings continuously for periods ranging from a few moments to several days, taking a single set of readings and assuming that they represent typical conditions, and having individuals wear small gauss meters that continuously measure exposures over time. None of these methods has yet won the support of the research community, however. Each has shortcomings.

The most reliable, albeit unproven, way scientists have for gauging EM field levels inside homes is a method called *wire coding* that simplifies the process. Wire coding estimates in-home exposures on the basis of the types of wires outside the home and the distance from the home to the wires. Because investigators have found a consistent association between wire-coding exposure estimates and some types of cancer—particularly childhood cancers—this method is very important, though it is not easy to apply on a house-by-house basis.

Skeptics of wire coding question whether the method accurately accounts for all EM field exposures and whether it represents some other agent or factor such as traffic patterns. They contend that the only way to correlate cancer to exposures is to measure the exposures using one of the other methods mentioned earlier.

Wire-coding supporters believe that the method is a better way to estimate EM field exposures over weeks, months, and years than measuring for short periods of minutes, hours, or days. Since EM fields vary widely depending on the amount of current flowing on the wires and other conditions, wire coding might provide a simple way to obtain average exposure information. Direct measurement methods seem to miss the subtleties of exposure, they say.

Because the wire-coding issue is pivotal and because you will hear about it often in the research literature, take a moment to understand how it works. (See page 161 for a more detailed explanation.) A physicist named Ed Leeper devised a system in the late 1970s to distinguish homes near distribution lines according to the amount of current the different distribution lines were carrying. Current, measured in amperes, or amps, reflects the demand for electricity, and it varies according to the type and number of electrical appliances that customers are using. If a family is using all of its appliances at once, it will consume a lot of electricity and the current will be high. If the family is asleep and only a few appliances are operating, the current will be low. Since the amount of current determines the strength of an EM field, the amount of electricity demand—known as the load—on a distribution line determines the EM field strength in nearby homes.

Leeper divided the homes he was studying into four categories according to the amount of current estimated to be running on distribution lines nearby and the distance between the homes and the lines. Leeper took sample EM field readings to fine-tune and confirm his method. He concluded that the method was reliable, and subsequent experiments seem to bear him out.

The reliability of wire coding is central to the EM field debate. In large-scale studies, exposure estimated by the wire coding method is consistently linked to cancers, while spot measurements are less reliable. The outcome of the debate will depend, to a significant degree, on the reliability of wire coding.

In your own life, wire coding may be useful if you live in a community where the distribution lines run above ground and you can "read" the power line configurations, although you may need help from your local utility to do so.

CRITICALLY EVALUATE WHAT YOU HEAR

In the early 1990s, utility companies from San Diego to Maine received a flood of requests from concerned customers for EM field measurements in their homes. As concern mounted, most utilities did the measurements but cautioned customers that they could not draw conclusions from the readings. This cautious utility response nonetheless represented progress from just a few years earlier, when company officials reassured customers indiscriminately that all EM field levels were safe under all circumstances.

At the same time, some activists used the accumulating scientific evidence to argue that the hazard had been established and that safety standards should be set. Many scientists and media observers accused them of fear mongering.

The EM field issue is tangled in a complex and high-stakes political, economic, and legal web. Almost everyone who has followed the subject closely has a stake of one sort or another in the resolution. That is why you should learn to think critically about what you hear. It does not mean that you can trust no one—only that you should consider all sides in a balanced way.

The utility industry historically has downplayed the significance of the research and the degree of concern among the public, while a small but growing number of activists play up both. The federal government for most of the past fifteen years has underestimated not only the research but also the level of public concern, and so has provided little guidance. But since 1990, that attitude has been changing slowly. In the absence of federal action, a few state and local officials have taken action, but these efforts are scattered and limited.

The net effect has been an information gap about EM fields and their possible health effects. A cottage industry has emerged to fill that need: EM field consulting and mitigation firms. The wide disparity in the accuracy and reliability of these services and products has further complicated the issue. Remember, no one is going to answer your questions better than you.

CHAPTER 3

PRACTICAL TIPS
FOR REDUCING
YOUR EM
FIELD EXPOSURES

Y OU CAN REDUCE THE LEVEL OF EM FIELDS YOU ARE EXPOSED TO
and the length of the time you are exposed. (Chapter 5
offers similar advice for EM radiation.) Since every home
and office is unique, however, you should use the suggestions here that make sense for you, your family, and your
co-workers.

The information in this chapter is organized in four parts.
The first addresses common appliances and electrical devices;
the second covers power lines and other external sources
(transmission lines, distribution lines, and transformers); the
third discusses wiring inside your home and workplace; and
the fourth helps you evaluate a house or an apartment, and
assess schools for your children, if you have any.

Use this information to survey and evaluate exposures
in your home and office. Try to understand the logic as well
as the facts so that you can make discretionary judgments
that fit you and your family. There are too many appliances

and electrical devices to cover all in this chapter, so I have included only the most common ones. That way you'll gain enough information to evaluate EM field conditions on your own. Simply follow two general rules: know your exposures; and be sensible in your responses.

Your first step should be to conduct a thorough survey of your home or workplace. Begin by drawing a simple map and marking electrical outlets on it. Add your electrical appliances and light fixtures to the map, trying to be as accurate as possible. Look for the circuit breaker or fuse box, and identify the thick cables coming into it. Follow these cables outside along your house or building, if necessary, and trace them back to the distribution wires that run between your home or apartment building and the electric power lines that bring electricity to you.

After you have completed the survey, retrace your steps and look for "hidden" sources such as fluorescent lights on the ceiling of a room underneath a bedroom. Remember that EM fields are present in all directions around a source. Try to envision those appliances, fixtures, and wires in close proximity to people but hidden behind walls. In particular, note where the electric lines outside your home or workplace are close to commonly used inside areas.

Pay particular attention to rooms where you have lamps or other devices that can be turned on by more than one wall switch, since these can suggest unbalanced circuits. If you have fuses rather than circuit breakers, the wiring probably is old and is likely producing higher fields than new wires would.

When you are satisfied that you have identified and mapped all your possible exposure sources, factor in your personal habits as well as those of your family or co-workers. If you spend a lot of time in one location, look at that place on your map. Could it be a high-field area? Could you reduce your exposures by moving your furniture? When you have questions about particular appliances, consult the lists that follow in this chapter. Do not assume that just because a device is small its emissions are low. A small, old-fashioned electric bedside clock can be a major source of exposure.

Whatever you learn from your survey and map, don't panic. EM field exposures are complicated and the net exposure conditions are not always what they seem to be. If you believe that a particular area of your home is a high-exposure area, there are steps you can take to confirm this and do something about it.

Your survey and map will help you make rough estimates. If you have identified an unusual situation, you can either get a meter to take measurements yourself or contact a qualified engineer to take readings for you. (See Chapter 2 for advice on measurements.)

Often it is simpler to make modest changes to insulate yourself from possible high-exposure conditions. The easiest thing, in many cases, is to move the EM field source farther from the area you are concerned about. Pushing your computer back on your desk or moving a laser printer into another room are easy ways to protect yourself. Sometimes it is easier to turn electrical devices off when you are not using them.

You also might consider rearranging furniture. If you cannot move the photocopier, perhaps you can put your desk on the other side of the office. If the distribution lines outside your home run along your child's bedroom, make sure that his or her bed is as far as possible from the side near the lines.

ELECTRICAL APPLIANCES AND DEVICES

Air Conditioners and HVAC Systems   Air conditioners consume a lot of electricity, and the high current flow can produce high fields. (This is one reason why magnetic field emissions from power lines generally are greater during the summer than during other seasons.) Large buildings that use industrial-size heating, ventilation, and air conditioning (HVAC) systems usually locate the equipment on the roof. Living and work spaces should not be located directly below the HVAC equipment. If they are, enclosing or shielding the equipment with a piece of magnetic field-reducing metal could be effective, but it will be costly.

Bedside Clocks   You spend six to eight hours a night near this relatively high-emission EM field source. The motors in dial-face clocks usually emit higher fields than do digital clocks. Most digital clocks emit lower levels, but do not assume they are low-emitters. Move either type of clock as far from your bedside as you can.

Calculators   Desktop calculators that plug into wall sockets use small transformers that emit magnetic fields when the calculator is on. If you cannot replace your calculator with one that runs on batteries, try to use one that has the transformer located on the plug (farther from the user). This type of transformer looks like a small cube.

Computers   See VDTs.

Desktop Task Lighting   Fluorescent task lights, like their ceiling-mounted counterparts, use ballasts that can throw off significant fields while the lights are on. Keep them at a distance. Better yet, use an incandescent light.

All halogen lamps—desktop and floor models—have transformers. The transformer commonly is situated in the heavy base of the desktop model or in the heavily weighted base of the floor model. Keep your distance from these transformers, as with all transformers.

Electric Blankets Don't use them, if possible. If you must, use a low-emission blanket designed specifically to reduce exposure. Conventional electric blankets produce fields as high as 300 milligauss within one-half inch of the surface, while low-emission blankets produce fields about twenty times weaker. Even though the magnetic field is eliminated when the blanket is turned off, the electric field remains as long as the unit is plugged in. At the least, use the blanket to "preheat" the bed, and unplug it before you get in bed.

Electric Heaters In some areas of the United States and around the globe where electricity is less expensive than other energy sources, electric resistance heaters are common. In addition, some people use portable electric heaters as small-area space heaters. Both types can produce modest, localized fields. If you are using an electric heater as a space heater, warm up the room before you use it, but run the heater for the least possible amount of time while you are in the room. Put the heater as far away from you as possible.

Electric Pencil Sharpeners The motors in these devices can emit strong EM fields when you use them. Use a manual pencil sharpener.

Electric Razors The bad news is that electric razors can emit high magnetic fields—up to 500 milligauss within one-half inch of the body of the razor—owing to their high-speed motors. One study has linked electric razors to cancer.

The good news is that few people use electric razors for long periods. Those that do—hair stylists and barbers—should consider traditional razors.

Fluorescent Lighting In fluorescent lighting devices, the bulbs are attached to a ballast, which is the major source of power frequency EM fields in many office buildings. Standard fluorescent office fixtures use four bulbs, each with its own ballast. As with ceiling fans, the exposure may be a greater concern for people on the floor above the lighting than in the room being lit, depending on whether the fluorescent fixture is suspended and, if so, how far. So your concern should focus primarily on the room below you.

Reducing these emissions is possible but not necessarily simple. Using an alternative type of electronic ballast virtually eliminates power frequency emissions but instead introduces very low frequency emissions in the EM radiation range. It is possible to arrange two sets of fluorescent light units side by side and head to foot, so that the emissions from each cancel those from the other. This may not produce the desired lighting effect, however. It may also be possible to purchase four-bulb fixtures with the cancellation arrangement already in place or to purchase one-bulb or two-bulb ballasts on your own and construct a low-emission fixture by arranging the ballast at opposite ends with the fixtures side by side.

Finally, lowering fixtures that are mounted on ceilings is an effective way to reduce field levels on the floor above. Be thoughtful when you do this, however, since lowering it also means that you are increasing the exposure levels in the room being lit.

Hair Dryers Use hand-held units at the lowest effective setting for the shortest possible period. Try to avoid using them for children's hair. In general, use a towel as often as possible.

Halogen Lamps In the base of most halogen lamps is a transformer, which adapts the electrical current from the wall socket into electricity that the halogen lamp needs. Like most transformers, these can emit significant but localized field levels that you want to avoid. Halogen lamps first gained popularity as desk lamps, bringing a new EM field source into the office. Manufacturers have also developed halogen area lamps and halogen bedside lamps. Both also use high-emitting transformers. In a few instances, the transformers are located in the plug unit for the lamp rather than in the lamp base. This usually makes it easier for you to be farther from the magnetic field source.

Laptop Computers Since laptop—or notebook or portable—computers do not use the same cathode ray tube (CRT) technology that desktop computers and TVs use, they do not produce power frequency and very low frequency emissions. The magnetic field from the computer's circuitry is minimal, since laptops are designed to operate on the smallest possible amount of electrical current. Laptop batteries and recharging equipment can emit weak fields, however, so you should not keep the laptop on your lap if you can put it on a desk or another surface. When you plug your laptop into an outlet, the plug consists of a cube that is, in fact, a transformer. Keep the transformer as far from you as possible.

Laser Printers Laser printers consume very little electricity while they are on but not in use, but when they are printing documents they draw a surge of current. The primary EM field source is the motor that drives the printer, and your first step should be to determine where the motor is located. The best way to do this is by using a gauss meter.

At a few inches from the motor, the magnetic field exceeds 100 milligauss. About six inches away, the field drops to between 5 and 10 milligauss. At a foot away, the field is less than 1 milligauss.

Shielding a laser printer is possible but prohibitively costly. Your best protection is distance—do not work within several feet of the printer for an extended period. Make sure that no one else works on the opposite side of any wall that a laser printer backs up to.

Light Boxes Light boxes have a sheet of opaque white Plexiglas suspended over a fluorescent light. Designers, paste-up artists, and photographers often use them to backlight their work so they can align design elements or so that they can see slides and transparencies clearly. The ballast for the fluorescent light (see Fluorescent Lighting) emits strong magnetic fields that are of particular concern because using a light box requires you to lean over it. Expect fields of 5 to 10 milligauss at distances of two to three feet, and fields above 2 milligauss as far as five feet away.

The ballast is the problem, and it should either be shielded (expensive) or moved to the plug end of the electrical cord, though this may violate electrical codes. Turn the light off when you do not need it, and work away from the light table when you can.

Light Dimmers These devices work by clipping off part of the electrical current and discarding it in the form of an EM field. If you have a light dimmer near your bed or any other location where you spend long periods, replace it with a regular light switch.

Microwave Ovens An electromagnet in the microwave oven generates the microwaves that heat food. Microwave emissions are regulated by the federal government, but it is possible for microwaves to "leak" through faulty door seals. You should test for leakage annually if your microwave oven is located in a spot that might allow regular, close exposure. Simple devices that detect leakage are available through many hardware and some kitchen supply stores.

Microwave ovens also generate substantial magnetic fields as much as five feet away from the transformer needed to operate the unit. In most homes the safest place to locate your microwave oven is on top of your refrigerator. This keeps it at least a few feet away from children and it prevents them from moving close to the microwave oven to watch food cook, an unwise habit. Adults should also stay clear of the microwave when it is operating.

Motors Electric motors produce magnetic fields, often at high levels. Motors are used in electrical devices ranging from bedside clocks to electric saws to children's toys. For small motors, you should try to stay at least a few feet away most of the time. Larger motors use more current and so produce stronger fields; try to stay as far away as is practicable. When thinking about motors, consider all the possibilities. Ceiling fans, for example, emit strong magnetic fields. The greatest exposure is likely to be on the floor above the fan rather than in the room that the fan is cooling.

A number of specialty manufacturing companies produce special metal shields that can reduce emissions, but the shields are costly. Unless your job requires that you be close to motors for extended periods—if you use electric tools, for example—it is difficult to justify the expense.

Photocopiers   The technology and electrical circuitry of photocopiers is almost identical to that of a laser printer (see Laser Printers). Exposure levels are, as a result, similarly localized to within a foot or two of the motor that runs the copier. Make sure that you work as far from the copier as is practical and never less than a few feet.

Postage Meters   The motors in postage meters can result in moderately strong magnetic field emissions. Postage meters should be kept on separate desks or tables so that one person is not regularly exposed.

Television Sets   In the late 1960s, the public was alarmed by reports that TVs were emitting potentially dangerous levels of X rays. Though this turned out to be true only for a small number of TVs with manufacturing defects and it led to new federal regulations, it is a different issue from that of EM fields.

TVs are like VDTs (see VDTs), except that very few people spend six to eight hours daily within a few feet of their televisions. Millions of people do that every day with their computers. Children may be the exception, and you should insist that your kids stay at least three feet from the screen. In fact, as with VDTs, the primary emissions from TVs are from the rear or the right side, but the extra distance is a wise precaution.

Typewriters   Electric typewriters produce fairly strong magnetic fields, including pulsed fields when the typing element sweeps from the right side of the page back to the left. Emissions are similar to those from photocopiers and laser printers—more than 100 milligauss within six inches, between 5 and 10 milligauss at about six inches, and less than 1 milligauss at one foot.

Turn your typewriter off if you are not using it, or move as far away from it as possible.

Vending Machines   A combination of the fields produced by the fluorescent lighting system used to illuminate these machines and the rest of the electrical circuits can commonly exceed 100 milligauss. If you are purchasing a soda or treat, you need not worry. But if your office or workstation has a wall in common with a vending machine, see if you can arrange your work space so that you are as far as possible from the vending machine.

Waterbeds   Small electric heaters keep the water temperate. They also produce modest magnetic fields. Most waterbed heaters are located underneath the frame, giving you a measure of safety in distance. Still, you spend one-quarter to one-third of your day in bed, and it would be better to avoid the exposure, if possible. Waterbeds for kids seem unwise.

Water Coolers   Do not put your office chair next to a water cooler, since the compressor emits moderately strong fields when it runs. Like much other office equipment, exposures through walls also are a potential problem.

VDTs   More than 50 million people use computers daily in the United States, with many millions of others doing the same in other nations. VDTs (video display, or computer, terminals) generate EM fields as a result of the current flowing through the units. Those that are based on cathode ray tubes (CRT) like TVs—that is, almost all desktop displays—produce very low frequency (VLF) fields as a by-product of the devices that ensure precise images on the computer screen. This same technology, with the same results, is used in TV sets.

The most extensive survey done of VDT emissions looked at both power frequency (ELF) EM fields and very low frequency (VLF) EM fields. Richard Tell, of Las Vegas-based Richard Tell Associates, did the measurements for the federal National Institute for Occupational Safety and Health. Tell found that VDTs do not add significantly to the power frequency EM fields present in most offices. VDTs can increase VLF field levels considerably, however. VLF is a form of EM radiation that research has associated with problem pregnancies. (See Chapter 1.) In addition, Tell found that seemingly identical VDTs can produce widely varying VLF emissions when their internal components are produced by different manufacturers. This is important to you if you are having measurements made in your office; you cannot assume that if you have tested one VDT you have tested them all.

VLF emissions are produced by a device called the flyback transformer, which is located in most VDTs at the right rear (as you face the screen). This means that the highest exposures are likely to occur behind and to the right of the display rather than in front at the operator's position. Evaluate your computer to see whether anyone works in the higher field areas. In many large computer processing centers—whether the work is processing checks or word processing—workers are arranged in rows. This means that most people are working behind another person's VDT, a situation to avoid.

Tell's survey also found that VDT EM fields lose their strength quickly over distance, more quickly than many other electrical devices. This is encouraging, for it means that reconfiguring the work space around VDTs need not require large spaces around each unit; twenty-four to thirty inches is generally considered safe.

Over the past three years, more and more VDT manufacturers have introduced low-emission displays. While a small number of companies that sell VDTs at deep discounts will continue to market them without low-emission designs, most major manufacturers now routinely comply with a Swedish standard issued to limit VDT emissions. Known as MPR2, "Test Methods for Visual Display Units," the Swedish standard includes both a method for taking power frequency and VLF emissions readings of both magnetic and electric fields and threshold limits for the emissions. The limits at 50 centimeters (about twenty inches) are summarized below:

Range	Magnetic Field	Electric Field
ELF	2.5 milligauss	25.0 volts/meter
VLF	0.25 milligauss	2.5 volts/meter

A Swedish union active in VDT health and safety issues has rejected MPR2 as too lenient and has called for stricter standards. SWEDAC, the Swedish government agency responsible for the standard, defends the standard as an engineering—not a safety—standard. It reflects what is reasonably achievable using current technology.

A panel of U.S. computer company representatives and other electric equipment manufacturers operating under the aegis of the Institute for Electrical and Electronic Engineers has adopted a similar but less stringent set of emissions limits.

You have two other options for reducing VDT emissions. Certain metals, commonly known as *mu metals*, can effectively shield magnetic fields. A small number of companies currently produce *mu*-metal inserts for VDTs, but the inserts are expensive.

The high cost of this type of retrofit led one researcher to compare the costs of installing power frequency EM field reduction devices during manufacturing versus adding the devices or comparable ones after the VDT was made. Sweden's Dr. Yngve Hamnerius found that a simple unit installed during production costs about $1 per VDT compared to at least $100 per VDT for most retrofit approaches.

You also have the option of choosing an external device that reduces magnetic field emissions. Screens that fit on the front of your computer monitor sometimes are sold with the claim to reduce EM fields, but in fact are not effective. An effective device is a metal band that clips on to your monitor and wraps around it.

Displays that do not use cathode ray tube (CRT) technology do not produce VLF fields. These include almost all flat-panel display devices, including liquid crystal displays (LCDs) and light-emitting diodes (LED). (See Laptop Computers.)

Telephones   The earpiece of every telephone has an electromagnet that can produce a strong but localized EM field alongside your head as a by-product of making the sounds you hear. The designs of some phones result in very little or no emissions, however. If you test the phones in your home and find one has a notably lower EM field level, use that phone in the busiest location. If you have a gauss meter, take it along when buying a new phone. If all other factors are the same, choose the model with the least EM field emissions. (See Chapter 5 for information on cordless and cellular phones, which emit EM radiation.)

Magnetic Resonance Imaging (MRI) or Nuclear Magnetic Resonance   MRI units create strong magnetic fields to develop an image of internal body parts. In some respects, they do what X-ray machines do, but they produce significantly clearer images. MRIs emit complex magnetic fields that should be avoided whenever possible (obviously not when you are the MRI subject). Medical professionals, including MRI technicians, should be in shielded rooms while the units are operating. In addition, MRIs consume a lot of electrical energy, suggesting that the network of electrical wires and cables may contribute to overall EM field levels.

Only a few years ago, MRI units were rarely seen outside of hospitals. Today they are more common, and individual doctors or groups of doctors sometimes set up their own MRI centers. This could mean that workers in nearby offices are being exposed to high magnetic fields. If you work near an MRI unit, even if you do not work with the unit, take magnetic field measurements.

Trains   A minority of electric trains and subway or metro systems—including, for instance, the New York City subway—use power frequency electricity. Most others use direct-current electricity. Scientists at the Environmental Protection Agency measured EM fields on one power frequency transit system in Maryland and found magnetic fields as high as 500 milligauss in the passenger compartment. If you ride a train every day, find out what type of system (power frequency or direct current) is used and take some measurements of your own. You may not be able to take personal action to shield yourself, but the owners of the train can redesign the electrical equipment to reduce passenger exposures. Electric utilities sometimes lease rights along train routes, or rights-of-way, to run transmission lines, adding to the exposure levels in trains running under those lines.

Even direct-current train systems produce power frequency EM fields in the passenger area as a result of electrical devices located under the floor. These and other EM fields can be "very intense," according to the Environmental Protection Agency.

Magnetic levitation trains are generally considered the trains of the future. These trains float on a magnetic field, reducing friction and enabling the trains to move more quickly than wheeled trains. An obvious concern is that the magnetic fields that carry the train also are present in the passenger area. The federal Department of Transportation has studied these fields and has reported that the exposure for passengers is moderately high, but that there appear to be viable ways of reducing the levels as part of the train design and manufacturing process.

Power Lines and External Sources

Distribution Lines   The familiar view of distribution lines is three wires strung along telephone poles in suburban neighborhoods. In most cities and a growing number of suburban areas, however, utilities are burying distribution lines. Their primary concern is eliminating unsightly wires, not reducing EM fields.

Burying distribution lines will reduce emission levels if the lines are properly phased and balanced. Engineers for several electric utility companies have devised ideal methods for burying these lines in metal pipes that contain a type of oil. Simply burying a wire is no guarantee that your exposure will be less than from a pole-hung line. The ground has no real ability to block magnetic fields; by lowering a conductor the utility may be increasing, rather than decreasing, your exposure by bringing the source closer to you. Utilities estimate that the cost of burying lines to reduce emissions ranges from five to ten times the cost of stringing lines on telephone poles.

Some utilities are starting to use twisted cables that wrap the three wires around each other as part of their distribution networks. This will almost always reduce net emissions to background levels.

You can usually recognize a high-current line as three wires that are relatively thin compared to other distribution lines. Often they are aligned so that you see three horizontal lines if you look up at them from the ground. In addition, more often than not you can trace the wire from your home or business to these high-current lines. In one out of every few houses, the drop-off appears to come not from a distribution line but directly from a transformer (see page 74). The transformers are needed periodically to step-down the voltage so that appliances and fixtures will work properly.

When low-current distribution lines, or primary distribution lines, are strung on the same poles as high-current lines, usually they are above the high-current lines. In many instances, they are the only electric power lines on the poles, however.

Distribution lines are not going to go away, so a primary concern in evaluating potential risk is to measure the distance from the lines to your home, particularly to the areas in your home where you spend the greatest amount of time. While the field levels at various distances can be calculated, sagging wires, tree branches affecting the wires, and other factors often make these calculations useless.

Farther is better than nearer. If the distribution lines are strung along your house and along your neighbors' houses, as they are in some neighborhoods in Philadelphia and other northeastern United States cities, the magnetic field levels are likely very high. Take measurements, if possible. Similarly, in some old towns and cities such as Alexandria, Virginia, houses are built very close to the street, with narrow sidewalks. Power lines strung on telephone poles situated on the sidewalks are, as a result, very close to many homes. In rural communities and some suburban neighborhoods, the distribution lines are separated from the homes by large distances. These lines rarely produce high magnetic field levels in local homes.

Distribution Feeder Lines   These wires connect your home to the local electric distribution system and bring electricity into your home. Make sure that your home is fed using "spun" wires—three wires twisted together. If you have three separated wires coming from the main lines to your house, ask your utility company to replace them. If the utility is upgrading its wiring network, as many are, it may agree.

Distribution Line Transformers   After electric power leaves a substation, it travels along primary distribution lines, which in turn drop the power off to secondary distribution lines. The drop-off requires a transformer, which changes the voltage of the electric current.

These transformers are essential for the distribution of electricity to homes and businesses. They come in many sizes and shapes, but perhaps the two most common are the cylinders that hang on telephone poles in many neighborhoods and the gray or green boxes in every fourth or fifth yard in relatively new housing developments.

The magnetic fields from both types lose strength very rapidly as they move away from the source. Though you should not camp under a pole-mounted transformer, you also should not panic because you can see one from your living room. Transformers on the ground are a concern when they are used as seats or when they are the congregation point for children. Both practices are unwise. In some condominium complexes, the transformers are situated unnecessarily near the homes.

In commercial settings, the transformers can either be large electric boxes in industrial parks or, in large office buildings, in basements or on part of an occupied floor. In one instance, in Madison, Wisconsin, workers in a building deduced that a transformer was in use nearby because the magnetic field emissions were strong enough to interfere with the images on their computer screens. If you are experiencing this sort of interference, there may be a strong EM field present. Transformers emit modest magnetic fields that lose their strength over short distances, but their presence can suggest that the wires running in or out of them are carrying high-current electric power that can contribute significantly to the overall field strength.

Identifying transformers is important but not always easy to do in high-rise buildings or industrial parks. If you have a gauss meter or hire an engineer to take readings for you, you probably will home in on transformers fairly quickly. Because they are not aesthetically appealing, however, they are usually hidden or disguised. In high-rise apartment buildings and office buildings, they are set up routinely inside closets or rooms that you might not even know are there.

Transformers can be shielded (at a fairly high cost), they can be moved away from people, or they can be inspected for improper wiring and, if appropriate, rewired to reduce emissions. In some instances, it is costly but effective to replace a single transformer with two transformers of approximately half the capacity and arrange the two so that their emissions cancel each other out.

Electric Power Entry Points Survey the outside of your house to learn where the feeder lines from the power company enter your house. In some instances, the lines are fixed to your house as they wind around to the entry point, where they feed into your circuit box.

In addition to checking to see whether the power company has used "spun" cable to bring electricity to your home, look for a grounding wire that connects either your electric meter or your circuit box directly to the earth. What you do not want to see is a wire from either unit to an outdoor water spigot or any other plumbing device, although this is a common wiring shortcut. This is easily corrected by having an electrician run the grounding wire directly to the earth.

Substations   Substations are in many ways large-scale transformers. They convert the high voltages used to send electricity over power lines to lower voltages that primary distribution lines can carry safely.

Substations can emit high magnetic fields, and their presence indicates that both transmission lines and primary distribution lines are nearby. They can be located anywhere. Many substations that once were sited in undeveloped regions now are encroached upon by residential and industrial development.

These substations are highly visible, comprising webs of wires and electrical equipment. Older substations often are enclosed in mature trees and shrubs, but a confluence of transmission and distribution lines usually leads to the facility, clueing you in to its whereabouts.

In urban areas, in high-rise office buildings, in office parks, and in industrial parks, it is not unusual for substations to be housed inside a building where they are hidden from view. For instance, Manhattan alone has more than fifty substations.

People living close to substations may be exposed to high field levels, as well as EM field pulses resulting from power surges. Paul Brodeur, in his book *Currents of Death*, has profiled the concerns of the residents of Meadow Street in Guilford, Connecticut, where seven adults and children developed cancers, in a cluster of cases near a substation.

It is virtually impossible to mitigate substation emissions

to a significant extent. Distance is your best protection. If you currently live or work near a substation, consider taking magnetic field measurements at various times of the day and over an extended period to weigh your risk.

Transmission Lines (High-Tension Lines, High-Voltage Lines) There are an estimated one million miles of transmission lines in the United States conducting high-voltage and very-high-voltage electricity. Long criticized as visual pollution, the lines and the towers that carry them have emerged as a focus of the EM field debate, even though more people are exposed to EM fields from distribution lines than from transmission lines.

There are more than fifty commonly used configurations for transmission lines—that is, more than fifty ways that utilities routinely string the wires on towers. Engineers choose different configurations for a host of reasons ranging from the capacity of the lines to the lay of the land. Only recently have they added EM field levels to the mix.

Several factors affecting magnetic field levels are the same as those affecting exposures from distribution lines: the amount of current, the relation of current-carrying wires to one another (for reasons of field cancellation), current balance, and the distance between the lines and the people who are exposed. One factor that is more often an issue with transmission lines is the use of single-circuit versus double-circuit lines. Double-circuit lines are two sets of three wires jointly carrying double the amount of electric power of one set. (Figure 1 shows two simple double-circuit configurations.) Measurements have consistently shown that double-circuit lines in proper phase and balance produce significantly lower magnetic fields at ground level than do single-circuit lines. (Figure 2 shows two simple single-circuit configurations)

Figure 1

Double-Circuit Configurations

**Horizontal
Double-Circuit
Configuration**

Circuit 1 ● ● ●
Circuit 2 ● ● ●

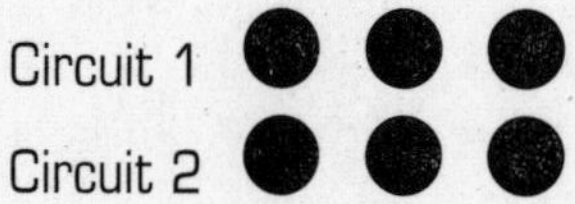

**Vertical
Double-Circuit
Configuration**

Figure 2

Single-Circuit Configurations

**Horizontal
Single-Circuit
Configuration**

**Vertical
Single-Circuit
Configuration**

Depending on configuration, phasing, and load balance, the emission levels can vary vastly. The Bonneville Power Administration, in Portland, Oregon, has found magnetic fields near or above 2 milligauss as far as 100 feet from a 115,000-volt line, 200 feet from a 230,000-volt line, and nearly 300 feet from a 500,000-volt line. You will need measurements to be sure of the levels in the area around the lines in your community. Delta configurations (see Figure 3) consistently produce the lowest EM field levels (assuming phasing and load remain steady across configurations), with double-circuit delta configurations (see Figure 4) the lowest of all.

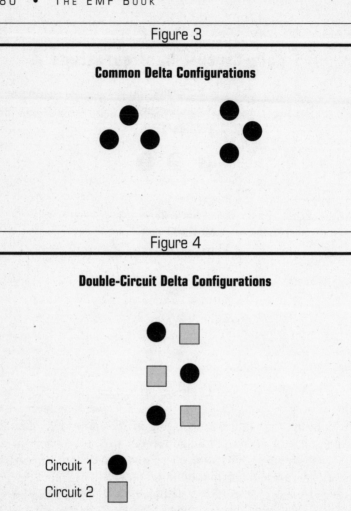

Figure 3

Common Delta Configurations

Figure 4

Double-Circuit Delta Configurations

Circuit 1

Circuit 2

Utilities have traditionally sited transmission lines where land is cheapest, which means that they are generally located where people are not. A combination of encroaching development in places such as San Diego, California, and rural western Pennsylvania and the need to deliver electricity in suburban and urban communities has pushed transmission-line disputes to the fore.

Of greater concern is the widely used policy of siting schools, playgrounds, and other municipal properties on or next to the corridors where transmission lines run. There are two reasons for this concern: First, obviously, schools are where we send our children and no one is willing to send his or her child to a place likely to be dangerous. Second, proximity to a transmission line coupled with the length of the school day means that schools near transmission lines are in conflict with two basic principles for reducing EM field exposures—distance and time.

Playgrounds and ball fields can be the center of social activity for children and adults, adding to their magnetic field exposures. Metal playground equipment can increase fields under certain circumstances, giving an ominous spin to seemingly harmless monkey bars and jungle gyms.

Municipal buildings are located on or near transmission lines because utilities have long been willing to sell property along the rights-of-way at greatly reduced costs. Not only does this put municipal workers at potential risk, but it is a model for what has turned out to be imprudent siting from an EM field perspective.

Many states and localities have proposed or implemented standards for EM field emissions from transmission lines, but they have had almost no effect on reducing exposures (see Chapter 8). The state limits uniformly are designed on the basis of engineering considerations and not at all on possible health problems. As a result they reflect levels at the edges of rights-of-way that most transmission lines already meet.

HOME AND OFFICE WIRING

Circuit Boxes or Circuit Breakers   Unless you are an electrician, you are not likely to spend long periods around your circuit box. Be sure, however, that your circuit breaker or fuse box does not back up on a wall near where you do spend a lot of time—for instance, the wall where the headboard of your bed is. Circuit boxes can emit fields of 100 milligauss or more, particularly when you are using peak amounts of electricity. If you are an electrician, be sure to work on a circuit box only when the power is turned off. This is wise anyway, as a way to avoid electrocution.

Internal Wiring   If you have an architect's drawings for your home or workplace, you will know where to look for wiring. Be forewarned, however, that electricians sometimes make changes in the wiring scheme. Do not assume that the architect's drawings accurately depict the way the wiring was done.

   To be certain where the wiring runs, you will have to conduct an extensive survey of EM fields using a gauss meter. How the wiring is grounded can also affect the field levels. Ideally, the circuit should be grounded by a wire running from the place where the electricity enters your home or building directly into the ground. Commonly it is grounded via a metal plumbing system at a point that is outside the house and that connects to the neighborhood plumbing system without entering the house. If the ground runs through the house via the plumbing it can produce a significant field inside your home. (Most homes built in the past decade use plastic pipes rather than metal ones, so this method is less common in newer homes.) Grounded current tends to run back to the electrical distribution system from which it came, seeking balance. This current can also contribute to the current on metal plumbing under some circumstances.

Certain types of wiring systems generate lower field levels than others. Improperly spaced wiring can cause high field emissions that are most easily found using a gauss meter. Karl Riley of Magnetic Sciences International, a Berkeley, California, firm, has reported that the magnetic field strength increases as the distance between the two conducting wires in an electrical system increases. For that reason, old-fashioned wiring systems that routinely left at least eight inches between the wires uniformly produce high fields. This is a concern only if your wiring is pre-World War II and it has not been updated.

Be alert to three-way switch systems that allow you to turn a device on from either of two or more switches. Wired properly, these circuits should not produce unusual field levels. It is not uncommon, however, for electricians to wire this type of circuit in a way that produces significant field levels. If the three-way circuit is in your family room, where you spend most of the time with your children, you need to correct the wiring. Low-voltage switches can further reduce magnetic field levels.

Once you have identified the areas in your home or office where the fields are higher or lower, use this information to determine how to lay out your furniture or work space. You may need to make use of an area that has a relatively high field level, so try to arrange the area so that you are there a minimal time. For example, put your filing cabinet there, not your desk.

House Wiring   (See also Internal Wiring.) Assuming the wiring meets accepted national codes, the levels within one foot of the wall can be about 3 milligauss and should not exceed 1 milligauss in the center of the rooms. These fields fall off rapidly. Since most furniture is within a foot or two of a wall, you should consider a magnetic field survey so that you can deduce where the wiring runs and identify any magnetic field hot spots—areas that you most want to avoid.

If the wiring does not meet code, the levels can be as much as ten times higher. A kind of wire cable called BX cable, which has spun wires in a steel casing, can help reduce field levels. More common Romex wiring can also be spun to reduce magnetic fields.

An easy way to determine whether the source of high magnetic fields is the internal wiring or an external source (for example, a power line) is to turn off the main power to your home at the circuit box. If readings in the center of the rooms remain high, the source is almost certainly external.

Taking a survey of magnetic field levels throughout your home or workplace is advised. Ideally, you should take a series of readings at different times of the day and on different days to gain a more complete picture of EM field levels. In particular, be on the lookout for hot spots—relatively small areas where the net magnetic field is notably higher than elsewhere—and avoid these spots. You may need to mark off high-emission areas if you find them at your workplace. Hot spots can be short-lived, depending on how you are consuming electricity, but more likely a hot spot will not go away.

Office Wiring   Offices with a lot of computers or other electronic equipment use scores or more of conducting cables to distribute power through the office. This can be done by raising the floor and running the cables underneath, or by running the cables through walls and other conduits. If you work in an office with a lot of computers (or even if the office next to, above, or below yours uses a lot of electronic equipment), these cables are likely to be a major EM field source. Do not expect to see them on an architect's drawings, though an architect or engineer may have added them if your office was remodeled recently.

Do not assume that your only exposure is from the equipment in your personal office—your computer, your desk lamp, fluorescent lighting, and so on. Scout out the offices next to yours, particularly on the side closest to your desk chair, as well as the offices below and above yours. High magnetic field emissions show up in unexpected places. Look for electrical closets containing circuit breakers, meters, and other equipment. If there is a locked door nearby that you have never seen anyone use, have someone open it for you. It may contain electrical equipment. If you work on the top floor of your building, find out whether there is an industrial-size air conditioning and heating unit or a transformer on the roof.

Your computer, a radio in your office, or a TV can help you determine whether your office has significant magnetic field levels. All electrical equipment can be affected by EM fields, a problem known as electromagnetic interference. In fact, the Federal Communications Commission regulates the type and level of emissions from electrical devices to limit this type of interference. Even a modest magnetic field can cause your computer screen or TV to blur or distort images and your radio to have poor reception. Other electrical devices, such as answering machines, may seem to malfunction.

REAL ESTATE AND SCHOOLS

Buying Real Estate When you or your attorney draws up the contract that you and the seller will sign, include a provision allowing you to test for EM fields as well as for termites, structural damage, and other major problems. Get an EM field survey done by a reputable tester or learn to do it yourself. Make sure the measurements you do are thorough—point of entry, plumbing, ground currents, appliances, light dimmers, and the like. If the property is vacant, you may need to arrange to have the power company turn the electricity on the day you do tests. Measure around the property. Look for distribution and transmission lines, and pay special attention to transformers. Is there a power substation nearby? Do your tests during a peak usage period, if possible, such as 7:00 P.M. or mid-afternoon on a hot summer day. You may want to ask the local power company to take readings, but do not rely solely on this information. You can also check with your state public utilities commission to learn whether the local utility has filed plans to construct any new lines near the property you are considering.

Have a licensed electrician check the wiring for possible violations of the National Electrical Code. Is the wiring properly grounded? How is it grounded? Ask the electrician to balance the loads at the circuit breaker or service panel. If necessary, get the local power company to replace separate feeder lines with a "spun" feeder.

If you are buying a home, take the time to visit local playgrounds and recreational areas, as well as the schools your children will attend, if you have children or plan to. Are there power lines near any of them? This could affect your decision.

Evaluating a School   If you have children, the first thing to look for in evaluating a school or one they may attend is whether the building or playground is sited near a transmission line, distribution lines, or a substation. As a precaution, the accessible area should be at least 150 feet from 115,000 volt transmission lines and as far as 400 to 500 feet from

765,000 volt lines. Measurements will help you assess a reasonable distance.

You can identify buried lines by the presence of electrical transformers—the gray or green metal boxes. Children often consider these boxes jungle gyms, so they should be fenced off at a distance of at least five feet. Measurements will determine the magnetic field levels from the buried lines themselves.

If there is metal playground equipment, take measurements in their vicinity. The metal can increase the net field exposures. Measure the field in various areas in the school at different times during the school day. Make careful notes about areas where you find levels that concern you.

Inside the school, first identify any major electrical power equipment such as transformers or electrical closets. Note their proximity to classrooms, lunchrooms, offices, and other regularly occupied areas. Try to determine from architectural drawings the routes used for electrical cables and wiring within the school, and take measurements to confirm the accuracy of the drawings. An electrician can determine whether the circuit for the whole school is balanced, as well as whether the circuits in individual classrooms are balanced.

Use the information provided earlier in this chapter to identify potential EM field sources. Rearranging computers or other electrical equipment may be the simplest and least expensive way to reduce field levels in the school.

CHAPTER 4

Your EM
Radiation
Exposures

W<small>E USE EM RADIATION ROUTINELY TO HEAT FOOD, TRANSMIT</small>
information, broadcast TV and radio shows, and measure
the speed and direction of cars, planes, and other vehicles.
Increasingly, we are using it to make telephone calls, communicate among computers in an office, and pay highway
tolls.

EM radiation also occurs from video display terminals
(VDTs), better known as computer monitors, and from TVs.
In fact, all modern electronic devices emit weak EM radiation
that we know can affect other electronic systems. Airplane
flight attendants ask passengers to turn off portable computers, tape players, and electronic games because these devices
can disrupt a plane's navigational equipment during takeoff
and landing. The Federal Communications Commission
(FCC) strictly regulates EM radiation emissions from consumer devices. Every electronic gadget you own had to meet
FCC requirements for electromagnetic interference.

This chapter will help you understand your exposures to EM radiation at home, at work, and in your community. We rely so extensively on EM radiation-based systems in our modern society that the first challenge is to recognize that products and equipment we take for granted may be EM radiation sources. Many people understand that cellular phones emit EM radiation, but they do not realize that cordless phones do, too. You may be wary of microwave ovens, but did you consider your neighbor's HAM radio transmitting antenna?

Equally important is knowing the difference between EM radiation emitters—or transmitters—and receivers. Satellite uplink dishes that TV stations use to beam their broadcasts to satellites for broad distribution emit radiation; satellite dishes on top of houses that pick up TV signals for home viewing are receivers. You do not need to worry about EM radiation from receivers, since there is none.

IMPORTANT FACTS ABOUT EM RADIATION

EM radiation is different in a number of key ways from EM fields. It contains more energy, and operates with shorter wavelengths and at higher frequencies. These characteristics give it the ability to penetrate the human body and to interact with molecules in unique ways. EM radiation at microwave frequencies (similar to those used for cellular phones) has a wavelength of about one inch, while EM fields at power frequencies have wavelengths of about 3,100 miles.

Scientists measure EM radiation in two ways:

1. The amount of energy emitted, described as the power per unit area, and expressed in watts per square meter (W/m^2) or, at lower levels, milliwatts per square centimeter (mW/cm^2). This is power density.

2. The amount of energy a body absorbs, expressed in watts per kilogram (W/kg), is known as the specific absorption rate, or SAR.

EM radiation can cause heating, so unlike EM fields you must be alert to possible thermal *and* nonthermal effects. EM radiation heating is not always immediately obvious to people who are exposed. For instance, radar repairmen accidentally exposed to thermal levels of EM radiation did not begin to feel warm until several minutes after the radar was turned on. Fortunately, most people do not experience this type of risk.

Radar and broadcast transmissions are very strong near their sources so that they can travel distances accurately and efficiently. For example, radar signals can be as strong as 7,500 milliwatts per square centimeter (mW/cm^2) at a distance of 750 feet. These levels will cause heating. In contrast, the EM radiation near the source of cellular phones is far lower—on the order of 1 to 2 mW/cm^2 at two inches. These do not produce heating and their health effects, if any, are nonthermal. Similarly, random EM emissions from electrical devices are extremely weak, though not too weak to affect other electrical devices.

Scientists differentiate between whole-body exposures and partial-body exposure. When the exposure strikes the body in just one area, that part of the body must absorb all the energy in the radiation. When the same amount of energy strikes the whole body, it is spread throughout.

EM radiation can be focused in a beam in a way that EM fields cannot. These beams can be broad or narrow, depending on their purpose. Microwave signals used to send telephone calls across a series of relay stations generally are focused, as the signals are aimed from station to station. Cellular phones send their signals in all directions at once, since the phones do not know where the nearest receiver is. Some EM radiation exposures concentrated in small body parts such as wrists and ankles produce hot spots. These hot spots also occur when a highly focused beam of EM radiation strikes a person. EM radiation also can induce strong electric currents in the body that can, in turn, reradiate. Both the currents alone and the reradiated—or scattered—radiation concern health investigators.

Two different EM radiation frequencies at identical strengths will produce different absorption rates in the same person, limiting scientists' ability to generalize across frequencies. EM radiation covers a very broad range of frequencies—roughly from 3,000 hertz (cycles per second) to 100 billion hertz. Not all of the frequencies are in use, but demand for available frequencies is growing rapidly. Until the early 1990s, the military reserved a vast range of the EM radiation portion of the electromagnetic spectrum. In 1992 and 1993, the government reclaimed many of these frequencies for commercial and industrial use, boosting the fortunes of the wireless age and markedly increasingly the amount of EM radiation we experience.

Health researchers have not begun to keep pace with the dizzying number of frequencies in use or the various ways that the frequencies are used. Every evaluation of your exposures must begin with recognition that research has taught us relatively little about specific frequencies and exposures, and most health assessments require assumptions across frequencies. It never will be possible to study every type of EM radiation at every frequency in common use.

EM radiation can travel long distances, and so we think of it in two parts: the near field and the far field. The near field is similar to EM fields. In the far field, however, the signal is clear and organized, making it both easier to measure and, in the case of a broadcast transmission, easier to convert into a TV or radio program.

EM radiation emissions are often modulated, meaning that engineers carefully design the signals to change wave shape in predetermined ways. AM radio is amplitude-modulated, for example, while FM radio is frequency-modulated. Engineers have developed increasingly sophisticated and complex methods of modulating signals to make better use of transmissions. Modulation can increase the amount of information a wave can carry, for instance. It also can change how an EM radiation signal might affect you. Researchers have found that modulation can alter the biological effects of a signal.

MAJOR CONSIDERATIONS

From your perspective, many of the guidelines described in Chapter 2 for thinking about EM field exposure apply to EM radiation exposure. You should seek to minimize exposure levels and limit exposure time.

For instance, avoid situations that could lead to EM radiation heating. If your job is repairing radar units, make sure that the safety procedures to ensure that the radar does not operate while you work are fail-safe. We know from experiments and accidents over the past sixty years that EM radiation heating can be harmful, even fatal.

For most EM radiation exposures, your concern is non-thermal. This means that you should presume that lower exposures are better than higher ones, even though there is evidence that lower is not necessarily safer. Until we know more, as with EM fields, the experts recommend you keep your exposures to the lowest possible levels.

The first rule is, of course, to keep your distance. Do not

work, rest, or play any closer to EM radiation sources than you have to. If you use industrial EM radiation equipment at work, try to configure the work space so that you will be as far as possible from the emitter while it operates. Remember that EM radiation travels better than EM fields, particularly as a focused beam, as with most satellite transmissions.

We can shield EM radiation more easily than EM fields, although it is not always simple or cheap. A conductive metal—such as a wire or a metal enclosure box—will convert the EM radiation into an electrical current. A grounded conductor will significantly reduce or eliminate the EM radiation signal. This is how consumer electronics makers usually meet Federal Communications Commission regulations for electromagnetic interference, for instance.

You also can reduce EM radiation at its source, though this makes sense only when the emissions are unintentional. A TV station wants to reach as many viewers as possible, so it will not intentionally weaken its signal. For computers and television sets, however, source reduction would not be counterproductive.

Measuring EM radiation generally is more difficult than surveying EM fields, owing to the wide range of frequencies and the complexity of the signals. It is possible to make broadband measurements, but they provide only limited information.

There are many EM radiation measurement specialists because of the demand for reducing electromagnetic interference. Most electrical engineers listed in your phone book can direct you to a qualified specialist, if he or she cannot do it.

With the exception of inexpensive (and generally imprecise) devices for detecting leaking emissions from microwave ovens, there are no commercially available meters for EM radiation readings. The sophisticated equipment that engineers use costs thousands of dollars.

Instead of comprehensive measurement surveys, you will have to use your new knowledge and some common sense. As Chapter 5 explains, you can identify most EM radiation sources easily and reduce your exposures most of the time by taking simple steps.

CHAPTER 5

PRACTICAL TIPS FOR REDUCING YOUR EM RADIATION EXPOSURES

Do NOT ASSUME THAT ALL YOUR EM RADIATION EXPOSURES ARE the same. Some exposures are environmental, some are occupational, some are optional, and the rest are at background levels. The lists in this chapter should help you evaluate and respond to those varying degrees of risk. You may want to avoid some devices altogether, while many others you might try to avoid when possible. A few may not concern you at all.

Exposures from such common sources as radio and television broadcasts should be low on your list of concerns, since it is unlikely they pose a significant hazard unless you live in a house among dozens of antennas. If you work near or with transmitters on a regular basis, however, you should view your exposures with greater concern. Finally, there are many devices that you could choose not to use, such as cellular phones and wireless baby-room monitors. Most of the time you do not have to give up these products, but you should learn to use them prudently.

The single most important thing to learn is how to recognize the variety and number of EM radiation sources. This chapter describes most of the common sources and offers practical advice on what you can do to limit or eliminate your exposure, where possible. As a rule, do not expect to eliminate all exposures. Every time you receive a radio station or make a cellular phone connection, you are exposed. That is okay.

Because EM radiation comprises so many frequencies and so many variations, and because the research is incomplete (see Chapter 1), you will rarely be able to directly match a specific exposure to a scientific finding. But while the jury is out (and it likely will be for some time to come), there are prudent measures you can take to safeguard yourself and your family.

ENVIRONMENTAL EXPOSURES

Throughout your day, common devices expose you to EM radiation—almost always at low, nonthermal levels. Most of these sources produce useful, often necessary, signals. You cannot avoid them, but you can make yourself aware of them and find ways to reduce your exposures.

Local Radio Networks The most common uses for these local area communications systems are emergency alert systems (e.g., police dispatches) and messenger systems. Some taxi companies and many courier networks use them, though cellular telephones have begun to replace them.

These networks require moderately powerful transmitters at the base office and at each location. People living or working near the base transmitting antenna—which often is located on top of the office—as well as drivers may experience above-average levels.

Transmitting antennas, often on small, metal lattice towers in industrial or residential areas, may indicate that a local radio network is headquartered nearby. Municipal or local officials should be able to tell you about the antenna if you are concerned: who owns it, what it is used for, when it is used, what frequencies it uses, and how powerful it is. If they can not, the Federal Communications Commission in Washington, D.C., can.

You do not want a station-to-station radio antenna near your workplace or home, if you can help it, because it will expose you almost continuously. If you live in an apartment building or work in a high-rise, check the roof of your building to see whether there is a broadcast antenna there.

Microwave Transmitters Microwave relay networks have replaced most of the old "wired" systems for sending telephone calls. Instead of routing telephone calls along wires, phone companies beam the calls across an extensive network of transmitters and receivers. Eventually, microwave relays will replace local calling connections as well. Often, these relay transmitters and receivers look like gray kettle-drums on towers. The microwave signals are weak but focused, and they need a "line of sight" to work. This means that nothing can obstruct the view between a transmitter and its receiver, so microwave relays almost always are visible above the treeline.

You can also see microwave relays on the roofs of tall office buildings and apartment buildings in cities, again because they are above most buildings and provide a line of sight. Usually, the relays do not expose building residents to EM radiation because their signals are highly focused. In some cities, however, lines of sight require threading the relay signal through tight spaces between buildings. People who work in these buildings at the height of the signal could be exposed.

A simple visual inspection will help you identify potential problem relays. Make sure that you are not directly between two relay sites. Microwave relays commonly are located on antennas used for transmitting several types of signals. If you see antennas with what you believe are microwave relay transmitters, do not assume that they are the only type of transmitter in use at that location.

Traditional transmitting antennas (long and straight) also can broadcast microwave frequency EM radiation for communications. These antennas do not rely on a relay network but instead transmit their signals in all directions at once, sometimes exposing people in offices below them.

Whenever you see an antenna, find out what it is used for, what frequency it operates at, how strong its output signal is, and when it operates. This information will be critical if you want to assess possible health risks.

Pagers   Most pagers that you clip on your belt or carry in your pocket are receivers only, so their proximity need not worry you. Pagers receive their signals through EM radiation broadcast from antennas. Pagers that receive messages in broad areas, such as anywhere in the United States, receive signals from satellites. The most sophisticated pagers transmit very weak signals periodically to let the paging network know where they are. Avoid this kind, if possible, or be sure to keep it in a briefcase or bag rather than close to your body.

Radio and TV Broadcasts   Radio and standard UHF and VHF television broadcasts consist of complex EM radiation that is very strong near the transmitters and that loses strength over distance.

In most places, broadcasters site transmitters as high as possible—on top of the World Trade Center in New York City and the Sears Tower in Chicago, for example, or on Mount Sutro in San Francisco. Remember that physical objects such as trees, buildings, and mountains absorb and reduce EM radiation, and high antennas allow the broadcasts to clear many obstacles. The height of the transmitter decreases the radiation strength at the ground, where people are most likely to be exposed.

People who work or live in skyscrapers such as the World Trade Center or on Mount Sutro are closer to the source. Indeed, surveys at the World Trade Center found very high levels in offices on the top floors. Mount Sutro, where exposure levels near homes also are higher than average, has long been the site of controversy.

In at least one city, Honolulu, broadcasters have located antennas directly alongside apartment and office buildings to preserve the visual beauty of Hawaii's vistas. As a result, transmitters beam signals directly into homes and workplaces. In a long-running dispute there, residents have reported toasters playing radio broadcasts, and EM radiation measurements have documented extremely high exposure conditions. Avoid conditions such as these, if possible.

Technicians who make their living maintaining and repairing radio and television antennas are constantly exposed to higher EM radiation levels than the general public. For many, the exposure is unavoidable. These workers should take work away from the broadcast sites when possible to reduce the duration of exposure.

Most broadcast sites are surrounded by "safe" zones that usually are fenced in. This serves two purposes. For the owner of the facility, it protects against theft and vandalism; for the public, it limits access to areas where EM radiation levels are unusually high and can even cause shocks and burns.

Many broadcast sites were established in unpopulated areas, but encroaching development has brought homes right up to the safety fence. People in homes within a quarter-mile of the broadcast facility (depending on the strength of the broadcast) should learn all they can about the types and levels of EM radiation produced at the site. Think seriously about the implications of buying or building a house near a broadcast facility, even though there is no proof that the transmitter is hazardous. Existing sites are likely to incorporate new types of transmitters, as the demand for wireless communications technology grows.

In most instances, radio and television broadcast towers can house multiple types of transmitters (microwave systems, land-mobile radio, etc.). In rare instances, including one involving a family in Santa Barbara, California, people live in houses on antenna "farms"—sites with multiple towers. There is no justification for allowing anyone to live among transmitters, since exposure conditions at these sites can pose potential heating hazards, not to mention possible nonthermal effects.

By the time radio and television broadcast signals reach most homes they are relatively weak. Your radio or television antenna picks up the signal because its internal circuits detect the appropriate signal and ignore all others.

Radiofrequency Fluorescent Light Ballasts   Less common than the ballasts operating at power frequencies (see page 62), radiofrequency ballasts emit modest EM radiation levels. (You may need to contact the manufacturer of your light fixture to determine whether it is a radiofrequency or power frequency type.) As with power frequency ballasts, the primary exposure will be to people working on the floor above the fluorescent lights, assuming the lights are ceiling fixtures. Because the ceiling itself will weaken the radiation strength—unlike power frequency emissions—the higher floor is at least partly shielded. In the room where the lights are being used, the radiation levels decrease to just above background levels at the height of an average person.

You may need help in determining whether the ballast is power frequency or radiofrequency, but in either case the same mitigation method applies. Radiofrequency emissions will cancel each other out as power frequency emissions will if you place an equal number of ballasts side by side with the ballasts at opposite ends (see also page 62).

Satellite Uplinks   Some of the earliest and most publicized public disputes involving EM radiation centered on large metal satellite dishes that news stations and other companies use to send information to satellites in orbit. The satellites, in turn, broadcast the information.

Satellite uplinks, as they are known, use strong, focused beams of EM radiation. Access to satellites is at a premium, so users often start sending information as soon as a satellite rises above the horizon and continue until it reaches the other horizon. Near the horizon usually are homes, offices, schools, and other publicly accessible sites, raising concerns about exposure.

As the number of satellites in space increases, many uplinks will have greater access to satellites and will not need to work near the horizon. As uplink dishes have become more sophisticated, they have gotten smaller and now use less powerful (but more complex) EM radiation. Mobile satellite uplinks are common, but not necessarily safer.

You can always tell where a satellite dish is aimed, since it moves to follow a satellite. Stay out of the way, since you never know when it is transmitting. In addition, keep clear of a 30-degree area on either side of the direction in which the dish is pointing, since the signal gets broader as it moves away from the uplink. Finally, when you identify an uplink dish, scan the horizon for public facilities (i.e., schools, hospitals) and for homes that may be in the line of the signal.

Toll Systems   A growing number of highway systems use electronic toll collecting for commuters. Small radarlike transmitters beam a signal into a lane of traffic to identify cars equipped with electronic identification cards or stickers. The signal reflects back to a device that "reads" the signal and charges an account prepaid by the car's owner.

These systems use nonthermal EM radiation, and most drivers go through electronic toll systems without stopping, at most a few times each day. The likelihood that the systems pose a hazard seems small, but the risk is optional for drivers. The price of avoiding the exposure, however, may be waiting in line.

Toll collectors working near the electronic toll system transmitters may be at increased risk, however, depending on how close they are to the radiation. The signal is focused, but broadly, and collectors in adjacent booths may be in the beam. Ideally, the electronic-toll collection transmitters should be in the outside lane so that the number of workers exposed is minimal.

OCCUPATIONAL EXPOSURES

Without knowing it, many people work with equipment and devices that produce EM radiation. In a hospital, for example, any health professional trained in the use of diathermy equipment understands that it uses EM radiation to produce heat below the skin for therapeutic purposes. Most health professionals probably have not considered that wireless cardiac monitors fill hospital wards with low-level EM radiation. Similarly, police officers know how their radar guns work, but few realize that it might not be safe to let the operating gun rest in their laps.

Awareness is important in the workplace. If you work with wireless communications devices, equipment with the terms *radiofrequency* (or *RF*), *microwave*, or *radar* in their name; computers; or any other system that relies on EM radiation, you should evaluate your exposures and consider ways to reduce them.

The following list of common EM radiation sources in the workplace may not cover your situation exactly, but it will give you basic information you can use to assess your own circumstances.

Computers   See VDTs.

Medical Equipment   As high-tech as most medical offices and hospitals are, EM radiation exposures are widespread. Medical technologies such as diathermy and magnetic resonance imaging can produce EM radiation at moderate levels. For the patient, these therapeutic devices hold more potential good than harm, but health professionals who are exposed regularly may want to be cautious.

Diathermy produces a highly localized exposure area, so occupational exposures should be minimal. Magnetic resonance imaging devices (MRIs) generate very strong and complex magnetic fields at low frequencies and also can produce some EM radiation. Though researchers have found only weak evidence linking MRIs to health problems among workers, they have completed too little research to assure us that MRIs do not pose a risk. MRI operators should stay as far as possible from the unit while it operates.

Wireless communications devices in hospitals can contribute significantly to EM radiation levels. More and more bedside monitoring devices—from heart monitors to fetal monitors—report to nurses' stations via EM radiation, saving the nurses and doctors valuable time and improving their ability to detect changes in patients. Since hospitals must plan and maintain these systems carefully to avoid interference, you can ask the hospital for detailed information about the operating frequencies and power outputs.

Surgeons and nurses working with electrosurgical units may be exposed to extremely high levels. Electrosurgical units are common operating room equipment, and at least one investigator has warned that a serious hazard may exist. Shielding these units is possible, though costly.

Police Radar   All police radar works in the same way, but there are two kinds of transmitters. The original transmitter sat on top of a police car or on a tripod outside a police car. Later, police departments mounted similar transmitters inside some patrol cars, usually on the metal cages that separate the back seat from the front seat.

For ease of use, police radar manufacturers found a way to put the transmitter in a hand-held unit, which we commonly refer to as a radar gun. To use it, an officer points it in the direction of an oncoming vehicle. Athletes and coaches also use these guns to gauge the speed of a pitched baseball or the velocity of a hockey puck. By measuring how rapidly the signal bounces back to a detector in the gun and the distance the signal travels, the unit can calculate the vehicle's speed.

When an Ohio state trooper named Gary Poynter observed what seemed to be a large number of his coworkers reporting cancer, mostly involving either the groin, the eye, or the brain, he began to wonder about police radar. He knew, as only a police officer would, that officers aimed cage-mounted radar units over their right shoulders and just past their heads. He also knew that for decades police departments trained officers to rest operating radar guns in their laps when they were not taking readings.

Even at just 1 millimeter from the transmitter, police radar units emit relatively low levels of EM radiation. The levels are well below thermal levels. So, while the possible cancer association is unproved, police departments have found that eliminating the potential hazard costs just $25 to $35. A simple device for mounting either radar guns or other transmitters on top of police cars virtually eliminates officer exposure without compromising the effectiveness of the radar devices.

Radar Radar uses EM radiation to take an electronic snapshot of a defined area in space. Since the area is usually large, radar units transmit strong signals.

Radar is used for a host of applications, but the three most common are (1) navigation and air traffic safety, (2) military observation and detection, and (3) weather observation and forecasting. Within this framework, different types of radar use different frequencies and send different types of signals.

Air navigational radar relies on a system of widely spaced radar units that measure speed, direction, and altitude. These large units generally are located outside metropolitan areas, but in many instances the population has spread out toward them. Workers at a radar site are unlikely to be exposed to high levels unless they are physically on or near the radar transmitter when it is turned on, which should be never.

Air traffic control radar systems at airports can expose

controllers and other workers to substantial EM radiation. Many airports have placed their radar systems on top of the air traffic control tower where the controllers work, and the broad beam can produce elevated exposure conditions inside.

Military radar comes in far too many models and types to catalogue all possible exposures. Those most likely to produce high exposure levels include shipboard radar systems from which avoidance is difficult if not impossible and airborne radar systems such as the AWAC planes that bathe themselves in strong EM radiation. These are flying radar stations, with large transmitters mounted on the planes.

As with other radar units, weather radar installations should not, under proper operating circumstances, expose any personnel to significantly elevated levels of EM radiation. The key factor with all radar is ensuring that it is operated properly, that it is not malfunctioning, and that precautionary safety procedures are followed strictly. Radar repairmen working on transmitters when their colleagues accidentally turned the unit on have been fatally injured—in fact, cooked much as a microwave oven cooks food.

If there is a radar unit in your community, particularly if it is a large one, or if you live near a military base, you should try to learn what the radar does, whether it is directional (focused) or omnidirectional, and whether the operator has established safety procedures for its staff. If the radar is used for military purposes, however, you may not be able to get this information.

RF Sealers   Drawing on the ability of radiofrequency EM radiation to produce heat, RF sealers melt plastic and other materials for industrial production. Vinyl three-ring notebooks are made with RF sealers, for instance.

A series of measurements in the late 1970s and early

1980s found that RF sealers in general expose their operators to high EM radiation levels. Some exceeded federal safety standards based on thermal effects, and many more approached the standard. Operated at torso level, the sealers expose operators—most of whom are women—to some of the highest sustained exposure levels ever measured in the workplace.

It is not possible to eliminate EM radiation emissions by redesigning RF sealers, but special clothing designed to reduce higher-frequency microwave radiation now is available for radiofrequency exposures. While the clothing has not been tested for RF sealers, you may want to learn more about it if you operate a sealer. (It was originally produced for radio and television broadcasters, so the best place to seek information is from your local broadcaster.)

Televisions   Televisions use the same technology as computer terminals, or VDTs, so they produce the same type of EM radiation, usually in the same areas. Fortunately, unlike VDTs, it is rare for people other than television repairmen to spend long periods behind a television.

Do not let children sit inches in front of a television, either, since even there the EM radiation from the set can be relatively high.

VDTs   In addition to producing EM field emissions, VDTs— for video display terminals—produce very low frequency (VLF) pulses that are one type of EM radiation. As a result, for much of the early 1980s, computer users expressed more concern about VLF emissions than about EM field emissions, though that changed as the scientific community showed increasing concern about EM fields.

As described in Chapter 3, VDTs can produce substantial VLF emissions, and seemingly identical VDTs can produce widely varying VLF emissions. You cannot assume that if you have measured VLF emissions from one computer you know what is coming from identical models. However, low-emission VDTs are increasingly common. Most major manufacturers routinely meet a Swedish standard released in 1991 (see page 69).

Flat panel displays do not produce VLF fields. These include liquid crystal displays (LCDs) and light-emitting diodes (LED). These may be practical alternatives, and several VDT manufacturers market their flat panel displays as "EM field and EM radiation safe."

Walkie-Talkies   Professional walkie-talkies (not the children's toys) operate near the frequencies that cellular phones use but with a higher output level. As a result of the publicity that accompanied claims that cellular phones might cause brain cancer, some people who use walkie-talkies are concerned.

Do not use a walkie-talkie if you do not have to, but recognize that they may be necessary in some circumstances. If you are foreman of a construction crew and you can answer a question in person or by telephone (but not cellular), choose that option. If shouting gets the job done as well, shout.

You can also tilt the walkie-talkie antenna (above the earpiece) away from you while you talk and back toward you while you listen. The transmission is greatest when you are talking, and this reduces your exposure, at least a little.

Wireless Local Area Networks (LAN)   Office computer networks traditionally have used wires, but wireless local area networks are easier to set up and easier to change, explaining why corporate spending on wireless LANs increased 158 percent from 1989 to 1993. The explosion in wireless LAN has brought with it a significant increase in the amount of EM radiation in the office.

If your local computer network is small or if you do not expect it to change significantly, stick with wires. If you work in an office with a wireless LAN system, arrange the office so that the transmitters are as far as possible from you and your co-workers.

Wireless Modems and Personal Digital Assistants (PDAs) Portable computers and their cousins, hand-held PDAs, created a fast-growing market for wireless modems (which transmit computer data). If you cannot wait to get back to a wired connection (such as a phone), move away from the wireless modem or PDA when it is transmitting data.

OPTIONAL EXPOSURES

Not everyone would agree that a baby-room monitor or a microwave oven is optional, but if you are serious about limiting your EM radiation exposures you should think of them as such. No matter how useful or convenient, some EM radiation sources are options that we could do without some or all of the time.

Alarm Systems Some alarm systems use EM radiation to detect motion, but since the radiation signals are weak and because they usually are in unoccupied areas, they are of little or no concern. In addition, alarm systems that signal either the police or a private sentry company in the event of a break-in usually do so with EM radiation signals. These signals are rare (you hope), most likely to occur when no one is around, and more beneficial than potentially harmful.

Baby Monitors   Few parents would argue with the practicality of portable baby monitors that reassure you your baby is sleeping and well. Still, there are two ways you can reduce your baby's exposures.

First, move the microphone—the part you leave in the baby's room—as far as possible from the baby's crib or bed. Baby-monitor microphones are very sensitive (most can pick up the sound of a baby breathing from across the room). The microphone unit also contains the transmitter, which sends out a signal strong enough to reach you as far as seventy-five yards away.

Second, consider a wired monitor. These contain equally sensitive microphones and even though you cannot carry the receiver with you on your belt, you can turn the volume loud enough so that you can hear it as far as a cordless monitor will reach.

CB Radios   The citizen band (CB) radio fad of the 1970s foreshadowed the wireless age, but CBs emitted much stronger signals. If you have a CB in your car or truck, leave it there but use it sparingly. CB radios pose no hazard when not in use.

Cellular Phones   Cellular phone use skyrocketed in the early 1990s, and industry analysts predict that its use will increase rapidly into the next decade. Yet concerns about a possible link between cellular phone use and brain cancer cast a shadow on that future. The industry was caught unprepared in 1993 by the public uproar that accompanied one man's widely publicized claim that his wife's cancer resulted from her use of a cellular phone. Attempts to reassure cellular phone users backfired when the federal Food and Drug Administration rebuffed industry assurances on safety, stating that "there is not enough evidence to know for sure, either way."

Cellular phones send moderately strong EM radiation signals in all directions from the antenna. These signals must find the nearest receiver that will relay the signal into the phone network. Most cellular phones can produce sufficiently strong signals to reach receivers several miles away.

Cellular phones can produce significant exposure levels in the brain since their antennas are within an inch or two of the head. If you must use a cellular phone, use it as little as possible; if you can, wait until you reach a wired phone. Use the cellular phone only for emergencies.

For car phones, locate the antenna as far as possible from passengers. Most car phone installers can put the antennas near the rear bumper. Indeed, many car phone companies now instruct installers where to place antennas for passengers concerned about EM radiation. If you carry a portable phone attached to a bag that contains the battery and antenna, put the bag as far from you and other people as possible.

New cellular phone technology is using a different type of EM radiation signal—digital instead of analog—and researchers who have evaluated the change fear that digital may increase the potential risk. Until we know more, however, follow the general guidelines for reducing cellular phone use.

In response to public concern, several companies have started selling EM radiation shields for cellular phones. These shields wrap around the phone antenna on the side near your head. They may actually increase exposures, however, since cellular phones increase power output as needed when anything blocks the signal.

Cordless Phones Cordless phones operate at different frequencies and use weaker signals than cellular phones.

Unlike cellular phone signals that must travel miles, cordless phone transmissions must only be strong enough to reach back to the phone base unit, which transfers the signal onto a conventional phone line. As a result, the fields they produce in the brain are lower.

Most people with cordless phones use them as their primary phones, since they are indisputably convenient. Instead, try to use wired phones whenever possible. If you have to be outside or move around, the cordless phone may make sense. If you can stay in one place, use a traditional phone.

Garage Door Openers Some, but not all, remote-control garage door openers use very weak EM radiation signals to activate the door. The instruction manual that comes with the opener will tell you whether it does. In any event, always aim the remote control away from people, and do not let children play with it.

Microwave Ovens Long a focus of concern, microwave ovens should not leak substantial levels of EM radiation unless they are malfunctioning. Federal laws require that microwave ovens be designed to block leaks, although this shielding is not foolproof. Relatively inexpensive leakage detectors are available that can tell you whether your oven is working properly (see also page 65).

Food cooked in a microwave oven does not retain the EM radiation. EM radiation is different in this way from ionizing radiation.

BACKGROUND EXPOSURES

All electronic devices emit very low levels of EM radiation—radios, telephone answering machines, televisions, computers, and so on. The Federal Communications Commission limits these emissions, and all consumer products have built-in EM radiation reduction.

There are a host of other EM radiation sources that rarely, if ever, create high-risk exposure conditions, ranging from tennis court electronic umpires to hand-held navigational devices that hikers use to pinpoint location. As you come across potential exposure conditions not mentioned here, consider the possibility that you are exposed to strong signals for extended periods. In most cases, you will find that you are not.

EM Field
and
EM Radiation
Policy

CHAPTER 6

PEOPLE
HAVE NEVER
BEEN MORE
CONCERNED

"Wow!"

U.S. Senator Joseph Lieberman said what many people in the hearing room seemed to be thinking. Are EM fields and EM radiation really as pervasive—and perhaps as hazardous—as the witness was suggesting?

Dr. Ross Adey, one of the world's leading experts on the biological effects of EM fields and EM radiation, was the star scientific witness at an August 10, 1992, hearing on the health hazards of police radar guns. An Ohio patrolman's informal survey and a series of news reports suggested that they might cause cancer. Lieberman wanted to know whether there were other possible hazards if, in fact, radar guns were linked to cancer.

Adey rattled off a series of commonly used devices that emit EM fields and EM radiation and that might be hazardous, including electric blankets, power lines, microwave ovens, and radiofrequency sealers, an industrial device that

117

seals plastic seams for products such as three-ring binders. He also mentioned hand-held cellular phones, which he added can "cause quite a high field in the brain."

The list was familiar to everyone involved in the debate over EM fields and EM radiation health effects. But in that hearing room on that day, when the question at hand was whether police officers were getting cancer while catching speeding drivers, the thought reverberated: *Maybe this stuff really is dangerous.*

People like you have never been more concerned—and confused—about the possible hazards of EM fields and EM radiation. News reports regularly warn that a new study has added to the evidence linking exposure to cancer, learning disorders, and other, more subtle hazards. Most people you meet have heard *something* about how power lines "cause" cancer or computers cause miscarriages.

Awareness that something is going on is at an all-time high. Public officials at the federal, state, and local levels now concede that the issue will not fade away, utilities respond to the issue daily, cellular phone companies have watched their stocks sink on mere allegations of a health risk, law firms have started a bidding war for experienced EM field and EM radiation attorneys, and the task of reducing exposures is expanding from a cottage industry to a substantial business.

It may be the environmental issue of the decade, bigger than asbestos; or a nonissue that has resulted from fear-mongering and junk science. Without question it is one of the most contentious and complex public health issues in history—one that analysts already compare to asbestos and cigarettes, for better or worse. What is certain is that this issue will not go away quietly. Nor should it.

The health-effects research is inconclusive but suggestive. Too many studies link EM fields and EM radiation to cancer, learning disorders, reproductive problems, and changes in body chemistry to think that the issue is a scientific fad. We are facing a period of scientific uncertainty and controversy that is likely to continue, at a minimum, into the twenty-first century. We live in an environment filled with EM fields and EM radiation, and escalating demand for electricity and wireless devices ensures that our electromagnetic environment will get more crowded, more complex, and perhaps—if this stuff really is hazardous—more dangerous.

WHY PEOPLE ARE CONCERNED

You may wonder how an issue can seem so important and yet so obscure. For more than a decade, study after study has linked EM fields and, less often, EM radiation to a range of health problems. Public attention has focused on cancer. Like a steady, slow drumbeat, the studies have attracted a curious public.

Since the first modern EM field study was published in 1979, research results have accumulated linking it to a few types of cancer in particular and all types of cancers in general. The results have been reasonably consistent—for instance, two independent research teams repeated the 1979 study and found similar results. Together they make a compelling cause for concern that EM field exposure can cause cancer in children living near power lines. Other studies in homes and workplaces show consistent, but not conclusive, links to brain cancer, leukemia, and male breast cancer.

Laboratory experiments using animals or animal organs indicate that EM field exposure changes some normal biological functions. These studies support the possibility that there is a cancer link and point to a variety of other effects, including learning delays, sleep disorders, and reproductive abnormalities.

For EM radiation the cancer link arises as well, though researchers have not studied it thoroughly. Laboratory studies have found subtle but significant changes at the basic level of cellular behavior and in the growth rate of tumor cells. For both EM fields and EM radiation, there are studies also showing no effect. Over time, however, the ratio of positive studies (which show effects) to negative studies has risen steadily.

During the late 1980s, public curiosity grew into concern. The scientists, and with them the media, seemed to get more serious about trends in the research. Several notable events marked this evolution, the first of which occurred in 1986 when a prominent scientist announced, to the surprise of electric utility scientists and lawyers, that he would buy a house farther from a power transmission line instead of one alongside the line if the houses were identical, even if the house near the power line were significantly cheaper. Though it did not makes national news, it was a warning to an industry that had been, until then, confident that EM fields was a nonissue.

The next major event came in 1989, when a widely distributed report to the congressional Office of Technology Assessment (OTA) gave public voice to the shifting scientific view. It reported that,

> As recently as a few years ago, scientists were making categorical statements that on the basis of all available evidence there are no health risks from human exposure to power frequency [EM] fields. *In our view, the emerging evidence no longer allows one to categorically assert that there are no risks.* [Emphasis added.]

In congressional hearings, in utility company boardrooms, in meetings of public utility commissions, and in countless living rooms, the OTA report set off alarms.

A year later, the staff at the Environmental Protection Agency recommended in a widely publicized report that EM fields be classified as "probable human carcinogens" (carcinogens are cancer-causing agents) and that EM radiation be considered "possible human carcinogens." The Bush administration then toned down the EPA's recommendations, sparking a public and media reaction that pushed the issue across the threshold from scientific pursuit to public issue. The major news networks and most of the national and major newspapers reported on the EPA document and on the subsequent White House role in altering the conclusions. Even if, as critics charged, the EPA recommendations overstated the mainstream thinking of the scientific community, the fact that scientists at the nation's top environmental protection organization had reached such a strong conclusion sent shock waves through the research community, state legislatures, and American industry.

One congressman reasoned that regardless of the White House changes the issue now deserved greater attention and caution. "There can be no doubt that power line EMFs have passed the 'duck test'; if it acts like a potential carcinogen, it must be addressed as a potential carcinogen," Representative Peter Kostmayer wrote to the EPA.

In September 1992, the Swedish government took what to many seemed to be the next logical step, deciding to act on the "assumption that there is a connection between exposure to power frequency magnetic fields and cancer, in particular childhood cancer." This called into question the view that governments everywhere lacked the evidence to act. Said one state health official, "The implications are just staggering in terms of protecting the public."

From the vantage point of a health-conscious public, the issue would never again be the same. In the wake of the publicized EPA findings and the Swedish decision, all EM field and EM radiation studies made news, and many reported cancer links. By January 1993, the Sunday magazine of *USA Today*, reported in a cover story titled, "Is My Electric Blanket Killing Me?" that its readers worried more about EM fields than any other environmental problem.

THE PUBLIC DEBATE

Until the late 1980s, scientists and policy makers had hoped that science would resolve the major questions one way or the other before the EM fields and EM radiation debate took on a life of its own. That hope is gone.

The rapidly increasing number of legal challenges to new power line and radio transmission towers are sometimes unfounded in science and law, but these lawsuits are pressing regulators and elected officials to develop policies for EM field and EM radiation safety in the absence of federal direction. Personal injury lawsuits may seem frivolous, but they have touched a nerve and confirm suspicions that the legal issues will continue to expand. Some utilities may be overreacting when they reassure the public with a level of confidence that research does not justify, but legitimate concerns about ensuring an adequate supply of electricity as well as liability implications drive their decisions. The cellular phone industry may be growing at a record pace, but the advancing wireless age raises troubling questions. Some of the devices and techniques for reducing exposures may be shams, but many specialists now believe that limiting unnecessary exposures makes sense.

These overarching legal and policy issues, as well as

major unresolved scientific questions, are not the immediate concerns most people have. People like you want to know how to assess whether you and your family are safe, but so much of the information is technical, confusing, and conflicting. If you think you are at risk, what do you do about it? And if you think EM fields and EM radiation are hazardous, what do you want your elected officials to do?

Identifying, measuring, and reducing exposure at home or at work is a growing aim for countless millions of people worldwide. For example, while serving as a U.S. senator, Vice President Al Gore asked the Environmental Protection Agency to take EM field measurements in his office. After a team of EPA staffers found high magnetic field levels near Gore's desk, he borrowed a gauss meter (the device that measures EM fields), took a short lesson in making EM field measurements, and surveyed his home. (As a young subcommittee chairman in the House of Representatives in the 1970s, Gore held the first congressional hearing on possible EM field and EM radiation hazards from consumer products.)

EM field and EM radiation policy can take many forms. You can take precautions; community groups can band together to block the installation of new facilities they believe are potential dangers; politicians can set exposure guidelines or call for more and better research; utilities can configure their power lines in ways that reduce EM field emissions; and police departments can mount radar devices outside patrol cars to virtually eliminate officer exposure.

This topic needs to take root in our collective common sense. Anyone who wants to understand the science, technology, and politics of this field can do so. Whenever a complex issue affects you personally, the mystique fades away. You figure things out that once seemed impossibly dense because you have to, as if your concerns were producing a dose of intellectual adrenaline.

Most people assume that only physicists, electrical engineers, and cellular biologists can understand EM fields and EM radiation. Discard that myth. You need to understand this issue because it affects you every day.

CHAPTER 7

THE POLICY GAP

THE PENNSYLVANIA PUBLIC UTILITIES COMMISSION RULED IN LATE 1993 that scientific research linking EM fields and cancer did not justify blocking startup of a transmission line in the southeastern corner of the state. There were two reasons to feel uneasy about the decision: the PUC had earlier refused to hear from scientific researchers who planned to testify that the evidence showed a link; and the PUC used a standard of proof that stacked the deck against the citizens' group that wanted the line stopped. As a result, the PUC's decision was a public disservice and a reflection of how far the EM field and EM radiation issue in the United States has veered from an honest discussion of the facts.

To be certain, the research is inconclusive. What it is not, however, is meaningless. If cancer is linked to EM fields and EM radiation at the low levels indicated in the research, a significant portion of the American public now spends part of each day in potentially hazardous conditions. Facing this possibility, there is a gaping hole in national policy that is largely responsible for the fear, frustration, and confusion that a growing number of individuals feel. A second impact of this policy gap, as courts and state and local legislators and regulators seek to fill the need for leadership, is economic. Never before have utilities felt so much resistance to new power lines or communications companies to new transmitters. The cost of these delays, which may or may not be justified, ripples through the economy, affecting all of us.

The government needs to face up to this issue, to acknowledge that the health research results are cause for concern, and to take sensible steps to address public concern. Public leaders—elected officials, utility regulators, government health specialists—who want to help put the EM field and EM radiation debate back on the track of science and reason first must talk straight about the issue. False assurances can be as damaging as scare tactics.

When public officials sidestep people's real concerns for their health, as the Pennsylvania PUC did and as federal officials have done for more than a decade, they spur frustrated and sometimes scared private citizens to seek legislative, legal, and public recourse. This adds to the legal and regulatory quagmire in which the debate is mired. Court rulings focusing on fear of EM fields, rather than on evidence of EM field risks, is one reason for the steady increase in legal claims. Unfortunately, federal inaction for most of the 1980s left an information and policy gap that lawyers, courts, and regulators are starting to fill. These efforts have caused confusion, delays, and hostility, and no one is winning.

There are alternatives to the Pennsylvania PUC approach (see Chapter 8 for more on legislative, regulatory, and legal actions). In Wisconsin, for example, utility regulators require electric power companies to consider steps for reducing EM field emissions from new transmission lines, and in California the state convened a working group comprising public officials, private citizens, and utility representatives to build a consensus on EM fields. In Sweden the government has decided to act on the presumption that EM fields are linked to cancer, and therefore to begin work on public safety standards for new power lines. At EM radiation frequencies, several municipalities have set broad standards to protect public health.

The U.S. government has almost no EM radiation research and policy program, save a congressionally mandated study of police radar and cancer, limited oversight of industry-sponsored research on the possible health effects of cellular phones, and classified military research.

The federal government's EM field research program, established in 1992, is well behind schedule and inadequately funded. More important, the way it is funded will undercut its ability to provide results without a conflict of interest. Each public dollar is being matched willingly, even eagerly, by a dollar from electric utilities, electrical equipment manufacturers, commercial electronic producers, and others with a direct financial and legal stake in the outcome of the research.

While the quality of research under this program will likely be high, the funding structure will raise questions about the credibility of the results, fairly or unfairly. Similar questions already have undermined tens of millions of dollars of electric power industry–funded research that has not been able to overcome public concerns about utility self-interest and allegations that scientific data is being manipulated, even though there is only circumstantial evidence on which to rest these claims.

Finally, the federal government should take the lead in promoting EM field and EM radiation awareness, in publicizing options for reducing exposures at home, at work, and in the community; and in encouraging new technologies that reduce exposures and perhaps risk.

Instead, since at least the mid-1970s the federal government has bobbled, dropped, and booted the ball. The federal EM field and EM radiation research and policy program historically has been severely fragmented, internally inconsistent, and unfocused. Initiatives started in the 1970s by the Federal Communications Commission, the Environmental Protection Agency, and the Occupational Safety and Health Administration to set practical federal safety standards or guidelines stalled at virtually every step, and then were simply abandoned during the 1980s in the spirit of deregulation and the de-emphasis on environmental and occupational safety that marked the Reagan administration. Unfortunately, as long ago as 1971, the Nixon administration warned that "the consequences of undervaluing or misjudging the biological effects of long-term, low level [EM radiation] exposure could become a critical problem for the public health . . . ."

Research programs—particularly the Department of Energy's—were neither creative nor aggressive. Where there was promising research, such as at the Environmental Protection Agency's laboratory at Research Triangle Park, North Carolina, the government simply shut down the facilities in the wake of budget cutting.

The Energy Department had far and away the largest government research budget on EM fields during the 1980s, but its primary mission is to promote energy production and delivery. It is not a health agency, and its half-century of work on the health effects of ionizing radiation has proved to be one of the federal government's most alarming debacles of the century. Not only did the department fail to protect the health of people working at its facilities where radioactive materials were produced for weapons, but it also knowingly injured hundreds of Americans in radiation experiments.

By late 1991, even top Energy Department officials agreed that the department lacked the credibility and objectivity to serve as the federal government's leading EM field research agency. In 1993, Congress reduced the department's role in federal EM field research and policy even though just one year earlier it had assigned the Energy Department the lead position. Congress named the National Institute for Environmental Health Sciences (NIEHS) to coordinate health research while the Energy Department oversees engineering and public communications work.

The Environmental Protection Agency, after losing its North Carolina laboratory, has gradually eased itself out of the EM field and EM radiation business. An EPA proposal to set forth guidelines for EM radiation exposures never made it to final form and simply disappeared from the agency's program. When Congress gave the agency $1.9 million for research in 1992, the nation's top environmental protection officials did nothing with the funds, even though agency staff had recommended a year earlier that EM fields be considered "probable" cancer-causing agents and EM radiation be treated as a "possible" cancer-causing agent. Even that groundbreaking report faded into oblivion. In 1993, the EPA virtually stopped all work on the incomplete project.

The Federal Communications Commission, with responsibility for much of the EM radiation portion of the spectrum, tried for a while in the mid-1980s to issue standards to protect the public from radio and television transmissions and other types of EM radiation. Even with strong public support from the broadcasting industry the FCC ultimately decided to do nothing. The industry feared that states and localities would set their own standards, creating a complex and inconsistent web of rules that would be far more costly and difficult than a single federal standard.

In fact, since 1992 the FCC has taken the lead to significantly expand the type and number of cellular phones, wireless office networks, and other consumer electronic devices that expose us to increasing amounts of EM radiation.

The Food and Drug Administration, which oversees consumer devices such as electric blankets, cellular phones, microwave ovens, and video display terminals, has been a passive monitor of federal inaction on both EM fields and EM radiation. Despite an occasional briefing paper or letter emphasizing that the federal government does not know enough to confirm or deny claims of EM field or EM radiation effects, the FDA has largely acquiesced to federal inaction.

With the increasing likelihood that trains of the future will ride on strong magnetic fields, as so-called bullet trains in Japan and Europe do, and with the realization that some subways and light-rail transportation systems expose riders and employees to high EM field levels, the Department of Transportation has shown interest in the research. By and large that research is primarily intended to help ensure the viability of a range of transportation systems.

The National Institute for Occupational Safety and Health (NIOSH), the research agency for worker safety, documented high EM radiation exposures for radiofrequency sealer operators—primarily young women—but never followed through on its findings. Radiofrequency sealers continue to operate today as they did in the late 1970s, when NIOSH first identified the problem. The agency's study of possible reproductive hazards associated with video display terminals (VDTs, or computer monitors) concluded with a misleading report that ignored valuable data the agency had gathered on VDT emissions at both EM field and EM radiation frequencies and reported that it found no link between VDT use and problem pregnancies.

The Occupational Safety and Health Administration, (OSHA), which is charged with setting rules for worker safety, tried half-heartedly to use a vague rule to regulate some EM radiation exposures. When a court said that the rule was unenforceable, OSHA officials simply abandoned it.

EM fields and EM radiation simply do not fit neatly into the federal bureaucracy, and no federal officials have stepped forward to figure out what to do with them. Instead, federal research and policy have wandered aimlessly and, by and large, unproductively.

At the White House, the Office of Science and Technology Policy maintains a committee to oversee and coordinate the disparate pieces of the EM field and radiation health effects policy-making system. The Committee on Interagency Radiation Research and Policy Coordination (CIRRPC) historically has functioned as the political hand to slow federal action. It was CIRRPC, through the Office of Science and Technology Policy, that pressed the Environmental Protection Agency to weaken its 1990 recommendation on the hazards classifications of EM fields and EM radiation. Indeed, CIRRPC issued a report on EM field research in 1992 largely to counter the EPA recommendations, broadly dismissing concerns that EM fields might be hazardous.

The many federal officials and agencies involved in research in the area responded with varying degrees of dissatisfaction to CIRRPC's report, with one exception. The report's "confirmation of the long-standing conventional view that commonly encountered EM field levels are not sufficient to cause adverse health effects is a reassuring conclusion," according to an official representing the Department of Defense.

The military, as the nation's largest user of EM radiation and a significant user of EM fields, has done more research than any other federal agency and perhaps more than all the agencies combined over the past fifty years. Much of the research remains classified, unfortunately. Several studies reporting positive results have leaked out, but the content and value of the remaining data are unknown. The military's steadily increasing reliance on EM radiation and EM field-based technologies for radar, communications, targeting, and even weapons (there is a class of experimental electromagnetic weapons), together with its considerable responsibility for national security, has turned the Pentagon's research program into an expensive rubber stamp. Results showing a health problem are viewed, unfortunately, as a national security problem.

Several authors of books and articles on EM fields and EM radiation health effects, including some who worked within the Pentagon's research program, have documented the military's long history of misrepresenting its research findings and of hiding key documents from public evaluation. In recent years, the military has organized letter-writing campaigns to discredit research and researchers it did not agree with and taken the hardest of hard-line stands against the possibility of danger from EM field and nonthermal EM radiation. The military's considerable influence in downplaying potential effects due to nonthermal exposures has only recently waned.

There are significant signs of change, even within the military research machine. Dr. Cletus Kanavy, the late director of the biological effects research team at the U.S. Air Force's Electromagnetic Effects Division, blew the whistle in 1993 on the military point of view. In an unusual document that accused another military official by name of scientific dishonesty, Kanavy succinctly summarized the volume of research that the Pentagon has historically ignored. Citing "new concerns" about EM fields at power frequencies, Kanavy warned that "the entire issue of human interaction with [EM] radiation is pushing forward as a major national population health concern."

That the federal government should take responsibility for EM field and EM radiation policy is indisputable. All interstate commerce such as electric power transmission and distribution and EM radiation communications is subject to federal authority. In situations where a patchwork of state or local rules might hamper this type of activity across state lines, federal policy always takes precedence. When the federal government does nothing, however, states and municipalities can act, though their authority may be challenged in court. Indeed, federal inaction has bred state and local action, which in turn has forced the federal government to act at last.

By spring of 1991, the utilities and the state regulators recognized that de facto EM field policy was emerging from the courts, from state and local regulators and legislators, and from utility responses to consumer concerns about possible EM field hazards. The number of lawsuits involving power lines has increased steadily since a Texas court ordered a Houston utility to pay a $25 million punitive fine to a school district for siting a transmission line across school property in "reckless disregard" of children's health. A small group of state officials, encouraged by utility leaders, met to form the National EM Fields Research Program (NERP) in June 1991.

At the time, more than a dozen states and municipalities were actively considering proposals to regulate power line EM fields, in addition to the growing legal docket. At EM radiation frequencies, cities such as Portland and Seattle were setting health-based restrictions on radio and television broadcasts, microwave transmissions, and other sources of public exposures.

No one seemed to understand the need for action at some level more clearly than John Coughlin, a public official charged with regulating electric utilities in Wisconsin who became chairman of the NERP. Coughlin argued forcefully for state officials to take charge if federal officials would not. In a speech that year, Coughlin explained that, "we can not wait until the science is clear. We are forced to make decisions."

Utility companies were finding it increasingly difficult to site new power lines and to add capacity to existing ones. State regulators in Pennsylvania, California, Florida, and Wisconsin were watching their proceedings backlog with EM field-based challenges.

The model for the NERP was another program created to resolve, in part, a power line dispute. In 1980, the New York Power Authority and seven other utility companies settled a long-running legal battle by agreeing to provide $5 million for a multiyear research project. The New York State Power Lines Project, completed in 1987, remains to this day the most important, comprehensive, and successful EM field research program. Contrary to the expectations of most of the people involved from the start, the effort not only confirmed prior evidence linking power line exposures and childhood cancer but found important new data indicating behavioral effects and other potential problems. The project's final report concluded that power frequency EM fields are a likely but unproven health hazard. The report also asserted that if a link between cancer and EM fields can be firmly established, then 10 to 15 percent of all childhood cancers are likely caused by EM field exposures.

Dr. David Axelrod, the Commissionor of Health for New

York State at the time, immediately recognized the need to increase EM field research at the national level. He sent the final report to federal officials. "As scientists and public health officials, we have no choice but to pursue responsible investigation of these questions, on a national if not an international scale," Axelrod wrote in 1987.

New York State officials expected their findings to jump-start the lagging federal research effort. From 1980 to 1987, while New York State ran a successful and highly productive research program on $5 million, federal spending estimated at $47 million between 1976 and 1991 had produced an effort that did little more than run in place. The New York State program produced the first confirmation of Wertheimer and Leeper's study linking power lines and childhood cancer, important new evidence that EM field exposures affect learning ability, and many other groundbreaking findings.

As a result of the multitude of promising leads the project had generated, New York State officials spent the years 1987 to 1991 planning and seeking support for what they informally called Power Line Project II. In congressional testimony he presented in March 1990, Dr. David Carpenter, who had directed the original Power Line Project, announced that the second phase was almost ready to begin. Eventually, however, Power Line Project II was transformed into the proposal that led to the NERP.

At a March 1990 congressional hearing, New York Power Authority's James Cunningham proposed a $15 million to $20 million program funded by electric utilities, with a board of national and state public officials and an independent scientific steering committee. Cunningham pressed the proposal with congressional staff members, with other utility executives, and with Bush administration officials.

Eventually, he found his way to a research group in Cambridge, Massachusetts, called the Health Effects Institute, or HEI. HEI had made a name for itself with a research program on auto emissions that was funded equally by the federal government and by the automobile industry. The organization was, at the time Cunningham first approached HEI director Andrew Sivak, working on an asbestos research effort funded jointly by asbestos companies and public sources. It was known as HEI-Asbestos Research, or HEI-AR.

The emerging structure for the NERP drew heavily on the HEI model, incorporating the public-private funding structure and the controversy that accompanied the appearance that self-interested funders might influence research results. The failure of the NERP steering committee and, later, Congress to eliminate this flaw burdened the resulting federal research program with a structure that will severely limit its value in resolving the health effects debate.

Sivak had positioned HEI effectively prior to the first NERP meeting on June 27, 1991. The Environmental Protection Agency had awarded HEI $525,000 to assess whether it could operate a research program such as the one NERP envisioned. Privately, an EPA official attending the meeting said his agency was interested in supporting the NERP only if the program were delegated to HEI. Most important, the NERP's model was HEI.

That should have set off alarms for the NERP steering committee. Steering committee members and their aides had grilled Sivak on charges that HEI-AR, the asbestos research project, presented at least the appearance of a conflict of interest. The charges arose from a resolution adopted by the National Association of Attorneys General (NAAG) that sharply criticized HEI-AR, including charges that HEI-AR had refused to address conflict-of-interest issues when NAAG had raised them.

Most electric industry representatives supported the NERP concept, though they all thought it premature to unreservedly endorse the NERP steering committee. They pressed the steering committee on its concerns about credibility.

Dan Shipp of the National Electrical Manufacturers Association, which produces equipment for the electric power industry, said that his organization had agreed in principle to provide $2 million to $3 million over five years for a NERP-type program, but that it was not prepared to make a firm commitment without a clearer plan of action. Shipp added that he was "uneasy" about the extended discussion of conflict of interest the previous day. Many top EM field researchers have received industry funding, he noted. "If you want a viable research program, you need to accept this and move forward," he said.

Cunningham had originally proposed that the steering committee include a representative of the Electric Power Research Institute (EPRI), a private nonprofit organization that conducts research on electric utility–related issues, including EM fields, with funding from the electric power industry. EPRI has spent more on EM field research than any other organization in the world, public or private, save perhaps the Pentagon. The NERP steering committee rejected the idea of including EPRI out of concern that it might adversely affect the group's credibility.

EPRI's role in EM field research was, and is, controversial. EPRI's critics contend that its overall research program is biased and, on occasion, that it has selectively chosen to follow up research that seems to downplay EM field risks and ignore its own research that points to health effects, and that it has misrepresented the results of projects it has funded.

Dan Dasho, an aide to Coughlin at the Wisconsin Public Service Commission, explained that, "No one on the Commission has a problem with [EPRI-supported] research," he said, "but every time you bring up EPRI research the public dismisses it." EM field activists tend to reject EPRI-sponsored research out of hand or discount it as biased. "If EPRI paid for it, it's suspect," says one activist.

Many scientists who have received EPRI funding forcefully defend the EPRI research effort. Granger Morgan of Carnegie Mellon University in Pittsburgh, Pennsylvania, backed EPRI at the March 1990 congressional hearing. "The main point," Morgan said, "is to keep in mind that EPRI is spending roughly twice what the largest federal programs are, and so while there may be problems of perception and otherwise, one also should not fault the industry for taking some significant initiative, which many others have not taken under similar circumstances."

Yet so polarized is the debate and so high are the stakes, that EM field research seems to demand a squeaky clean approach. The confusion, anger, frustration, and costs associated with the public health debates over agents as diverse as cigarette smoke, asbestos, and pesticides can be avoided only by a stringent conflict-of-interest policy that raises research results above suspicion.

The NERP was a reminder of the basic problem in setting EM field and EM radiation policy: the research data were insufficient to make clear policy decisions. Individual citizens, a growing cadre of EM field activists, and, increasingly, elected officials were arguing that the data justified mandated safety measures until research proved EM fields benign. From a public health perspective, from the economic viewpoint of the utilities, and from a prudent public policy standpoint, the proper way to solve this dilemma was to do more research and to do it as quickly as possible. Cunningham of the New York Power Authority, speaking on behalf of a consortium of about twenty large public utilities (known as the Large Public Power Council), warned that delays meant trouble:

The LPPC members, as I am sure all utilities, businesses, and individuals who have had to deal with this issue agree, believe it is absolutely essential that this study begin soon. Public opinion polls show that public awareness and interest in this issue is growing. They also show that they expect clearer answers from us in 2 to 3 years. Unless we act, this interest could quickly turn to heightened concerns dominated by emotions. History shows us such an environment is not conducive to good public policy. Facts do not penetrate emotions.

As the NERP steering committee proceeded, its commitment to avoiding conflicts of interest faded. Using funds raised from utility companies in Wisconsin and from the New York State Energy Research and Development Authority, the steering committee selected Energetics, Inc., a Columbia, Maryland, consulting firm to provide administrative support to the committee.

Energetics already had a contract to help guide the Department of Energy's EM field program, raising troubling questions about the ability of the firm to treat each client's interests separately. Considering its duties at the Energy Department, Energetics was in the position of advising government officials on decisions that directly affected the NERP steering committee, and vice versa.

The troubling situation was not lost on Representative James Scheuer, a congressional subcommittee chairman. At a 1992 hearing, Scheuer cautioned Coughlin that he had "noted with some concern" the steering committee's hiring of Energetics.

The Energetics controversy lost some of its importance in August 1992, when Congress formally designated the Department of Energy as the lead federal agency for EM field research. Department officials hastily scheduled an

interagency meeting for November 20 and 21 to begin planning a national research strategy that would, for the first
time, integrate diverse EM field research activities in various
federal agencies.

Energy Department officials pursued their leadership role
with a vengeance. The November 20–21 meeting, organized
by Energetics, was unprecedented for the breadth of interests
represented and for the demeanor with which the department
led it. Michael Davis, a senior Energy Department official,
conceded that "not enough has been done [by the federal
government] to satisfy questions about possible health
effects." Added Robert San Martin, yet another department
official, "it is time to mobilize and become more pro-active."

Energy Department officials either could not or would
not make a commitment to seeking more research funding,
however. "It seems unlikely to me that there's going to be a
massive injection of new federal funds," one said, irking several researchers. Mindful of the effort of the NERP steering
committee, federal participants from several agencies pri-
vately suggested that a public-private co-funding approach
could significantly increase funding.

In 1992, while Congress was approving $6 million for
Energy Department EM field research for fiscal 1993, Rep.
George Brown of California, chairman of the Science, Space,
and Technology Committee, led a successful effort to create
a multiyear national EM field research program modeled on
the NERP and using joint funding from federal and nonfederal sources. The program moved through Congress as part
of the National Energy Strategy Bill that President Bush
signed into law in October 1992.

The Brown program provided a total of $65 million over
five years—up to $12 million per year for EM field research
and up to $1 million per year for public information and
communications. Half or more of the research funds would

be reimbursed to the government by nonfederal contributions, so that the program would in essence use the same type of joint funding that the NERP had considered.

Congress set a very tight schedule for the federal National EM Field Research Program, but by mid 1993 the program already was well behind schedule. The interagency committee, charged with developing a research agenda, was not yet in place by midyear, and a congressional mandate to start research by January 1994 was missed. The Clinton administration made appointments to the advisory panel in late March 1993 that included John Coughlin and two other state representatives, one EM field activist, one labor union official, one scientist from the National Academy of Sciences, and two utility representatives. The group selected Shirley Lunde, the EM field activist, as its chairwoman.

In September 1993, following the first meeting of the advisory group, Chairwoman Lunde told *EM Field News*, a newsletter published by a utility group, that the new federal program that was set up to jump-start federal research already was well behind schedule and that such a delay might mean,

> we may not be able to get the answers that this program was created to get. We don't want to be in a position of having to go back to the American people with the same lament—that we need more research before we can provide any concrete answers.

The program's slow start, typical as it is of almost every other federal EM field research initiative, may be only the second biggest obstacle the federal National EM Field Research Program will face.

From the perspective of EM field activists and concerned consumers, there will always be a reason to question the credibility of research results from the federal program. In courtrooms in the late 1990s, plaintiffs' attorneys will use the issue of utility funding to raise doubt among jurors. In legislatures and regulatory hearing rooms, politicians eager to stand up for their worried constituents will exaggerate the role of the industry's support. Given the already murky political atmosphere in which EM field-related decisions are made and the high probability that the political air will get murkier during the next decade, it is difficult to envision how the federal research effort will achieve the type of credible-beyond-a-shadow-of-a-doubt standing it will need to significantly improve our nation's ability to make policy based on science rather than politics and emotion.

The virtual absence of an EM radiation research program certainly ensures that currently unresolved issues, as well as new concerns likely to arise as wireless technologies proliferate, will fester. And while the federal government stumbles, the legal, legislative, regulatory, and political landscape at the state and local level will get rockier.

CHAPTER 8

POLICY IN
THE MAKING

Some situations involving EM field and EM radiation exposures are easily within your control, such as whether you use an electric blanket and where you put your microwave oven. Many other situations are more complicated, such as when a utility company seeks to use some of your property to site a transmission line or when your job requires you to use equipment that emits EM radiation. These are the situations that most often lead to legal action, legislation, regulatory proceedings, or safety standards. There are circumstances in which you may want to act to correct what you believe is a past wrong, which is what happens when police officers sue police-radar makers because they believe the radar units caused them to develop cancer.

It is always easier to file a legal claim than it is to prove its validity. Getting a legislator to introduce legislation is relatively simple, while getting the bill signed into law can be difficult. Convincing a utility regulatory board to evaluate

public concerns is common, but establishing a generic policy for public exposures to EM fields or EM radiation is rare.
Challenging plans for a new facility is increasingly common,
while blocking the siting of an emitting source such as a
power line or a microwave transmission tower is more difficult, though not uncommon.

The federal government has, as Chapter 7 describes,
done very little by way of establishing clear policies for EM
field and EM radiation exposures, generally leaving that
authority to state and local regulators and legislators. Where
these officials either do not act, or act in a way some people disagree with (which is often), people file suit.

Outside the United States, there are exceptions. Sweden
has been more aggressive than any other nation in setting
safe exposure limits for computer users, and is working on
EM field standards for power lines. Japan, Poland, Russia,
and the United Kingdom all have adopted EM field standards, but the levels they use are far above what research
suggests may be hazardous. Canada and several other countries have adopted safety standards for EM radiation,
although these standards tend to reflect the view that nonthermal effects are not hazardous.

In addition, a U.S.–led group of industry and military
officials have created a voluntary standard based on thermal
exposures for EM radiation. Known as the ANSI standard, for
the American National Standards Institute, these limits are
used almost as often to justify the use of EM radiation sources
as they are to protect public safety. The ANSI standard also
serves as the basis for international EM radiation standards.

Two leading EM radiation research groups in the United
States have set much stricter EM radiation exposure limits
than ANSI. The Applied Physics Laboratory at Johns Hopkins University and the Phillips Laboratory at the U.S. Air
Force's Kirtland Air Force Base in New Mexico set maximum

worker-exposure levels that are approximately 100 times lower than those permitted by ANSI.

Seven states—Florida, Montana, Minnesota, New Jersey, New York, North Dakota, and Oregon—have established standards for EM field limits at the edge of the rights-of-way that surround transmission lines. These standards are "engineering" rather than "safety" standards; this means that they reflect the levels now common at most transmission line sites rather than limits based on health research. Several states, including New Jersey and Montana, have taken less specific approaches to limiting potential public-exposure levels. California has rules mandating minimum distances between power lines and schools.

Following a series of reported cancer clusters at schools in places like Fresno, California; Montecito, California; and Boca Raton, Florida, a national EM field and EM radiation advocacy group set its focus on reducing exposures at schools in all fifty states. As a result, numerous states surveyed the siting of their schools in relation to power transmission lines, and many found that a relatively high number of schools are located near the lines. In 1993, U.S. Representatives George Miller of California, the chairman of the House Natural Resources Committee, proposed legislation to put a 2 milligauss limit on EM field levels in all schools.

In the past, it was common for utilities to seek school property for their lines because this reduced the need to negotiate with individual property owners. School boards often welcomed the income. In addition, in at least some states, utility companies offered property near transmission lines to local officials for schools, municipal buildings, and playgrounds. Property along rights-of-way has long been less desirable than other property because most people do not want large industrial towers near their homes.

The EM fields and schools initiative has led a handful

of utilities to voluntarily reduce exposure conditions by reconfiguring or moving their lines. New York State utilities reached an agreement with the state attorney general in 1993 to measure exposure conditions in all schools near power lines. Some utilities are mindful of the landmark 1986 legal decision in which a Texas court ordered a Houston utility to move a transmission line sited across a school's property and to pay a $25 million penalty for siting the line in "reckless disregard" of children's health. At a small but growing number of schools, administrators are closing classrooms with high EM field levels or roping off areas in playgrounds where the field levels are unusually high, such as near metal playground equipment.

School officials also have permitted EM radiation sources on school property, though this is meeting opposition. Late in 1993, for example, the San Francisco Unified School District placed a ban on communications antennas on school property after a company proposed siting a low-power transmitter on one school. With tens of thousands of similar transmitters in use in the United States, an unknown number of them on or near school property, the issue is likely to receive increasing attention. A handful of schools have questioned the presence of cellular phone towers, for example.

Regulatory challenges to plans to site cellular towers and other EM radiation sources on a variety of types of private and public lands are increasingly common as well, though few are successful. At least two cities—Portland and Seattle—have standards in place to control EM radiation exposures.

Citizens who have asked regulators to disapprove utility companies' applications to site new transmission lines or to upgrade existing lines have similarly found success elusive. In Bucks County, Pennsylvania, Dottie English and other citizens in an affluent suburb of Philadelphia succeeded in forcing the state's Public Utilities Commission to reopen a proceeding. Philadelphia Electric Co., the utility company seeking to operate a new transmission line along an abandoned railroad right-of-way that bordered on a string of backyards, had completed construction of the line by the time the PUC issued its ruling, finding that there was insufficient evidence to justify blocking use of the line.

One of the concerns in the Bucks County case was that presence of the line would lower property values. Courts have, in the past, ordered companies to compensate property owners for lost value. Property owners have had limited success in these cases, though many realtors believe that EM field and EM radiation concerns are affecting sales. A 1992 cover article in *Real Estate Today* magazine warned that "concerns about power lines loom over sales."

One of the most important cases yet decided allows property owners to sue for lost property value because they believe their property values are hurt by the *fear* of EM fields—so-called cancerphobia—regardless of whether the scientific evidence provides cause for that fear. The case, involving a major transmission line across part of New York State, did not result in a payment to the property owners, however. It merely allowed them to return to court to sue for lost value. Courts in three other states—California, Florida, and Kansas—have reached similar decisions.

In rare instances, lawsuits, regulatory rulings, or citizen actions have blocked new lines or required reconfigurations of existing ones. A Michigan-based group forced a utility company there to abandon plans for a major transmission line intended to deliver electricity to Indiana. The group relied on congressional pressure—Michigan congressman Howard Wolpe held a hearing in the state and subsequently announced his opposition to the line—lawsuits, regulatory pressure, and media attention to delay the line until the utility threw in the towel.

A major battle was shaping up in Pennsylvania over a line planned to run across much of the state to delivery electricity to New Jersey. With more than 9,000 sets of written comments on file and citizens groups from across the nation vowing to make this a high-profile test case, the project died unexpectedly in late 1993 when a New Jersey court ordered a New Jersey utility to pull out of the deal for non–EM field reasons.

In Alexandria, Virginia, where the historic Old Town attracts powerful federal officials nightly from nearby Washington, D.C., a group of citizens successfully pressured city officials to reduce field levels in homes by moving, burying, or reconfiguring lines. The distribution lines in Old Town were just a few feet from many homes, and field levels inside the homes were consistently high.

Claims for personal damages have resulted in a mixed lot of decisions. A highly publicized case in San Diego, where parents of a young girl sued because they believed that EM field exposures from power transmission and distribution lines while the girl was *in utero* caused her to develop a rare form of cancer, resulted in a victory for the utility company. It was the first-ever jury decision for a personal injury claim involving power lines.

Police officers who have sued police-radar manufacturers claiming that exposures from the radar devices caused them to develop cancer have lost. More than a dozen police officers have filed suit, and none has won or successfully settled a case. EM radiation suits generally are more difficult than EM field suits since there is less available research.

An exception is the case won by a satellite technician who was accidentally exposed while working on a rooftop near a satellite dish. A judge ruled in favor of the worker, who suffered visual damage, when the company that owned the satellite failed to show up in court.

Several other EM radiation cases have resulted in out-of-court settlements. A one-time radar technician in the U.S. Navy won more than $130,000 for cataracts, and the widow of a man who died owing to what his family said was exposure to EM radiation received more than $150,000 from RCA. Other settled cases have involved radio and television broadcasts.

The largest award ever received also came about as the result of a settled case rather than from a jury decision. Robert Strom, a former Boeing Company employee who developed leukemia, received $500,000 from the company, while the company also agreed to pay for a medical program to monitor and treat other employees who, like Strom, worked in the company's electromagnetic pulse (EMP) program. In the settlement, the company maintained that the EMP was not hazardous. EMP is an extremely powerful burst of energy produced when a nuclear weapon explodes; the federal government has long studied it because of concern that it could generate a surge of current that would ruin most electrical equipment.

Strom used part of his settlement to set up a foundation that is encouraging others exposed to EM fields and EM radiation to file suit. As a result of his case, a team of lawyers has formed the Electromagnetic Radiation Case Evaluation Team to work together on EM field and EM radiation lawsuits.

Another notable case involved a woman who developed brain cancer, allegedly as a result of using a cellular phone. The case drew unprecedented media attention in January 1993—the woman's husband appeared on, among other shows, *Larry King Live* and the *Today* show. The attention caused cellular phone company stocks to lose value rapidly, though their prices recovered quickly. It also prompted the cellular phone industry to launch a public relations blitz, promising among other things to fund a new generation of research at cellular phone frequencies. The industry apparently did not take its promises seriously enough for federal officials, and key EM radiation specialists at the Food and Drug Administration later reproached the industry's trade group for its cavalier attitude to the research.

Instances where states proactively attempt to set EM field policy are rare but not unknown. Wisconsin was the first state to establish a policy of reducing EM field exposures from power lines, where possible. "It is reasonable to conclude that reducing exposure to [EM fields] increases public safety," the state's Public Service Commission ruled in 1992. "Doing nothing, while waiting for conclusive evidence about human health effects, is not a reasonable response to the potential risks associated with [EM fields]." Earlier in the year, the PSC had ordered Wisconsin utilities to use the "best available" technologies to reduce EM field exposures as part of their siting and planning processes.

Colorado was the second state to adopt a policy aimed at limited public exposures where possible at a reasonable cost. That state's Public Utilities Commission ordered utilities to include "prudent avoidance" in its planning, siting, construction, and operation of transmission lines. "Until scientific findings are more conclusive," the PUC ordered, "facilities should be designed and located using methods to mitigate, to the extent practicable, involuntary exposures to the public."

The next state to act was Connecticut, which took a significantly less aggressive position. Rather than requiring utility company changes, a state EM field task force recommended what it calls Voluntary Exposure Control, which it explains as "a pro-active program of providing information to the community about EM fields and factors to consider if concerned individuals decide to reduce their exposures."

POLICY IN THE MAKING • 151

California completed a years-long consensus-building process involving concerned citizens, public officials, utility representatives, and health specialists by setting an interim policy urging utilities to reduce "unnecessary" EM field exposures from new transmission lines so long as doing so does not cost more than 4 percent of the total project budget. The state's Public Utilities Commission issued the rule, but decided to postpone a decision on whether to reduce emissions on existing lines.

Massachusetts has an EM fields task force, but has not issued rules. In 1986, the state promulgated the broadest EM radiation exposure limits for workers then in use. The limits were based on the ANSI limits.

State and municipal activity is sure to increase at least until the federal government sets preemptive policies. In addition to the myriad legislative, regulatory, legal, and voluntary activities described here, scores of state and local legislatures are weighing exposure limits of various sorts. The number of lawsuits is rising steadily, fueled by the steady pace of new research results and increasing awareness among lawyers that this issue is not going away. Unless and until we accumulate a much more thorough understanding of EM fields and EM radiation and their effects on our health, the patchwork of policy initiatives and court rulings will grow, becoming even more of a problem for the delivery of electricity and information, and continuing to cost all of us who consume these two commodities more and more money, and perhaps our health.

Resources

APPENDIX A

A GUIDE TO EPIDEMIOLOGICAL RESEARCH

THERE IS A WEALTH OF RESEARCH ON HEALTH EFFECTS ASSOCIATED with EM fields and EM radiation at levels too low to cause heating, but there is considerable disagreement about the value of this evidence. The epidemiological data discussed in this chapter strongly suggest that EM fields play a role in cancer, but exactly what role and how large a role remain unknown. The data on EM radiation are far more limited but are cause for concern.

From an epidemiological perspective, EM fields are much easier to study than EM radiation for two reasons: First, EM fields involve just one frequency (60 hertz) or, at most, a very small range of frequencies from one type of source (the flow of electric current); while EM radiation involves millions of frequencies from a wide range of sources. Second, it is much easier to find a large group of people regularly exposed to EM fields (from power lines, for example) than to identify a large group regularly exposed to a single type of EM radiation.

The laboratory evidence discussed in Chapter 1 clearly indicates that EM fields and nonthermal EM radiation can cause biological *changes* at the cellular level and can affect the ways that cells communicate and interact at the most basic levels.

Still, researchers have not yet found a sufficiently clear and consistent pattern to reach a consensus on health effects. They are not likely to for at least another five to ten years.

This appendix is a reference to help you understand the epidemiological research. For most people, epidemiological studies and the statistical methods involved are daunting and confusing. This compilation, which is not available anywhere else in a nontechnical format, tells you only as much as you need to know to grasp the key points about a study or a set of studies; it combines statistical data and historical perspective. One of the most frustrating things about EM field and EM radiation research is that its complexity and diversity make it difficult to distill. This appendix will help.

As you read the study summaries, keep in mind that there are at least three ways to interpret the results: the scientific way, the public policy way, and the personal way. Scientists need unambiguous, confirmed data. Policy makers tend to take action on the basis of inconclusive evidence. You must decide what's best for you and your family.

These distinctions are important to the EM field and EM radiation debate. Policy makers, including elected officials, appointed regulators, and judges and juries are already implementing policy decisions on the basis of the incomplete data that we have. People like you are trying to make decisions on your own.

To do this, you should have at least a basic knowledge of the research that has been done. You can use the information in Chapters 2 to 5 to guide your decision making, but in our rapidly changing EM field and EM radiation environment you may need to refer to the science behind these recommendations.

Each study summary includes a citation that you can use to locate the original study paper, if necessary.

EPIDEMIOLOGICAL STUDIES

An epidemiological study attempts to gauge the probability that a particular agent—in our case, EM fields or EM radiation—is causing a particular disease by looking at patterns of disease among humans. The epidemiological method is to gather detailed data about a large number of people and then to make a series of comparisons between either (1) a group of people who have the disease they are studying (cancer) and those who do not have it, or (2) a group of people who have or are presumed to have EM field exposures in common and another group with little or no exposure.

In the first approach, called a *case-control study*, you try to match someone who has or had cancer (the case) to one or more people who does or did not have cancer (the controls). You can then compare elements of their respective homes, lives, personal habits (for example, do they smoke?). You can compare either the rate at which cancer occurs or the rate at which people die from cancer. These are called, respectively, *incidence* (or *morbidity*) and *mortality*.

In the second approach, known as a *cohort study*, you identify a large number of people who meet a criterion—for example, people who work in jobs that are believed to involve unusual EM field exposure conditions. For your cohort group, you select a larger and more diverse population (all the people who live in the city). If you observe important differences, you might be able to reach a conclusion about whether the exposed group is at greater risk of developing or dying from cancer than the cohort group.

Another way of doing a cohort study is to compare the rate of disease or death among your study population (the exposed group) to the rate you can expect to see based on national, state, or international statistics. These are known as either a *proportional incidence study* (when you are evaluating the number of people diagnosed as suffering from cancer) or a *proportional mortality study* (when you are comparing death rates). This approach is often an initial one, used most commonly to generate hypotheses that more sophisticated research can test.

None of these studies can produce "proof" that EM fields cause cancer or other health effects. Epidemiological research is based on statistics, and statistics describe probabilities, not certainties. Only in the very unlikely event that you have an extraordinarily clear result that different researchers successfully replicate repeatedly under a variety of circumstances without fail will you be able to say with confidence that a given agent causes a given health effect.

Smoking cigarettes causes lung cancer, and the human immunodeficiency virus (HIV) causes acquired immunodeficiency syndrome (AIDS)—these are two examples of research-established causal relationships. Remember that these relationships are statistical, and there will always be a minority of scientists contending that the links are not proved. Even with the most compelling evidence, some doubt will always remain. The data on EM fields and EM radiation are not nearly as conclusive as the research on, for example, smoking, asbestos, or pesticides. So if you are waiting for an unequivocal cause-effect conclusion, don't hold your breath.

There is a scientific convention that a study finding should not be "associated" with an agent unless you can use statistical tests to conclude that nineteen times out of twenty the result did not occur by chance or as the result of some other risk factor. If the association passes that test, the finding is "statistically significant." This is a *positive study*.

There will always be some people with cancer, most of the time with no clearly identifiable cause. These cancer cases are said to be chance events. In science, you want to be reasonably confident that your research results are not due to chance. In scientific studies, this probability is described by a *p-value*. Generally a p-value of 0.05 or less (1 in 20 or less) indicates that the result is statistically significant.

So it is that in EM field research, as in other areas of research, it is not unusual to come across studies reporting increases in the incidence of cancer, say, where the author concludes that his study is negative because the result fell short of "significance." The 0.05 value is not magic, however, and when you are reviewing scientific literature you should not ignore a study with a p-value of 0.049, for instance. If you had a string of experiments with p-values between 0.048 and 0.051, that should catch your attention.

The following guide to key epidemiological research is presented as simply as possible. Where it is appropriate, the summary includes explanations of how and why a study is important. This appendix is not all-inclusive; it focuses on the most significant studies and results—both postive and negative. The appendix is divided into two parts: EM field studies and EM radiation studies. It separates EM field studies into four categories: childhood cancer studies, adult residential cancer studies, adult occupational cancer studies, and reproductive effects studies. The EM radiation section includes cancer studies and reproductive effects studies.

EM Field Studies

Childhood Cancer

Childhood cancer is, and should be, a major concern of both public health specialists and the public. Leukemia, in particular, is the subject of intense interest because it is the most common cancer in children.

The possible link between EM fields and childhood cancer grew from the unexpected 1979 finding of researchers Nancy Wertheimer and Ed Leeper (see first study described). It has remained a lightning rod in EM field research not only because of its scientific interest but also because it resonates with the fears and the emotions of every parent. In a modern world full of magnetic field exposures, research suggesting a connection between these fields and cancer in our children will always be cause for concern.

Combined Childhood Cancers

Study authors: Wertheimer and Leeper
Date Published: 1979
Study type: Case-control
Reported Outcome: Positive

This landmark study set off the current debate with its finding that children who lived in homes near high-current distribution lines were approximately twice as likely to develop childhood cancer as were children living in other homes. The study included 344 children nineteen years old or less who died of cancer after living in a home near a high-current line, and an equal number of controls.

The study was not intended to evaluate whether EM field exposures cause cancer in children. Rather, the investigators set out to learn whether 344 children who died of cancer in Denver between 1950 and 1973 had anything in common. In the process of doing the research, Wertheimer noticed that a disproportionate number of the cases' homes seemed to be located near electrical transformers, the cylindrical metal devices suspended from telephone poles periodically along power distribution routes.

Further investigation revealed that the transformers appeared to be markers for high-current distribution lines. Leeper and Wertheimer did a series of measurements to confirm this. To facilitate the study, which would have been prohibitively expensive had they taken measurements in and around every house, Leeper developed a system for coding houses according to the type of distribution wires nearby. Almost fifteen years later, this wire coding scheme is pivotal to the scientific debate, and so it is worth explaining.

Leeper grouped homes as either high-current configuration (HCC) or low-current configuration (LCC). HCC homes met *one* of the following criteria:

- They were within 130 feet of thick three-phase primary distribution lines.
- They were within 130 feet of at least six thin primary lines.
- They were within 65 feet of three to five thin primary lines.
- They were within 50 feet of thin secondary distribution lines that had not yet delivered electric energy to any homes and that ultimately delivered energy to at least three single-family homes.
- All other distribution wire configurations were classified as LCC.

The investigators did enough sample measurements to be confident that the wire coding was a reliable surrogate for actual measurements at every home. They also recognized that because magnetic field strength is a result of the amount of current flow, the EM fields in and around the homes would vary widely in the course of a day and across seasons. Perhaps wire coding would turn out to be more than a useful surrogate for actual exposures; perhaps it would prove to be a more accurate way of gauging prolonged exposure.

Wertheimer, N and Leeper, E (1979). "Electric Wiring Configurations and Childhood Cancer." American Journal of Epidemiology 109: 273–284.

Study author: Savitz
Date Published: 1988
Study type: Case-control
Reported Outcome: Positive

This study was designed to test the results of the 1979 Wertheimer-Leeper study, and it confirmed them. Savitz concluded that EM field exposures estimated by Leeper's wire-coding system were associated with all types of childhood cancers. He also found a statistically significant link between wire coding exposure estimates and brain cancer in children. Actual EM field measurements taken at a sampling of homes were not associated with childhood cancer, although Savitz found a nonsignificant increase of cancer cases among children who lived in homes where the measured fields exceeded 2.5 milligauss.

Savitz studied 320 children younger than fifteen who had died of cancer in the Denver area between 1976 and 1983. He used 259 other children as controls. As part of the study, Barnes and Wachtel thoroughly tested the accuracy of the Leeper wire coding method and concluded that it was a reliable surrogate for EM field exposures.

This study was, according to Dr. Leonard Sagan, the top authority on EM fields for the Electric Power Research Institute, "A landmark study, one that established the EM field-cancer issue as deserving further attention."

Savitz, DA, Wachtel, H, Barnes, FA, et al. (1988). "Case Control Study of Childhood Cancer and Exposure to 60-Hz Magnetic Fields." American Journal of Epidemiology *128: 21–38.*

Study author: Tomenius
Date Published: 1986
Study type: Case-control
Reported Outcome: Positive

This study compared childhood cancer at 716 homes of children who died of cancer to 716 homes without childhood cancer deaths. Rather than assessing individual children, the study compared homes to see whether the exposures differed between case homes and control homes. The deaths occurred in children less than nineteen years old between 1958 and 1973.

Tomenius evaluated exposure levels in two ways: (1) he considered the distance between the house and 200 kilovolt transmission lines, substations, transformers, electric railroads, or subways; and (2) he took spot magnetic field measurements at the front doors of the houses. Overall, the magnetic field levels at the case homes were no higher than those at the control homes.

The study found, however, that the case homes were more likely to be within 150 meters (about 490 feet) of a magnetic field source. Tomenius also reported that the risk of childhood cancer deaths was twice as high in homes where the measured magnetic field was at least 3 milligauss. Both findings were statistically significant.

Tomenius, L (1986). "50-Hz Electromagnetic Environment and the Incidence of Childhood Tumors in Stockholm County." Bioelectromagnetics *7: 191–207.*

Study author: London
Date Published: 1991
Study type: Case-control
Reported Outcome: Positive

One of the most thorough studies completed to date, this investigation looked for associations between childhood cancer and both measured EM fields and EM fields estimated using the Wertheimer-Leeper wire coding method. It confirmed the findings of Wertheimer and Leeper (1979) and Savitz (1988) that childhood cancer is associated with wire coding–based estimates, but it did not find a link between childhood cancer and actual EM field measurements.

London and her team evaluated 232 cancer cases that occurred between 1980 and 1987 in children ten years or younger, and an equal number of children who had not developed cancer. All the children lived in Los Angeles County, California. Children living near high-current wires, under the wire coding system, were about two and a half times as likely to develop cancer as were other kids. This finding was statistically significant.

For measured fields, there was a 50 percent increase in risk for children exposed to the highest EM fields, but this was not statistically significant. Oddly, children with the lowest measured exposures seemed to be at greater risk than were those with exposures in the middle range. This type of inconsistency could signal a problem in the methods used in the study or indicate a probability that the seemingly positive finding—that is, the 50 percent, nonsignificant increase among the highest exposure group—is an anomaly. Other researchers asked whether wire coding is a better way of averaging or estimating long-term exposures than measurement. London used a limited number of twenty-four-hour to seventy-two-hour measurements but generally relied on much briefer measurements.

In an unexpected finding, London reported that children exposed to EM fields from black and white televisions (but not color ones) and from hair dryers had a statistically significant increase in cancer risk. The investigators concluded that this finding was "difficult to interpret" since the duration of appliance use (including TVs and hair dryers) was based on the recollections of parents. Past recall is generally considered less reliable than real-time observations, though it is commonly used.

London, SJ, Thomas, DC, Bowman, JD, Sobel, E, Cheng, TC, Peters, J (1991). "Exposure to Residential Electric and Magnetic Fields and Risk of Childhood Leukemia." American Journal of Epidemiology *134: 923–937.*

Study author: Myers
Date Published: 1990
Study type: Case-control
Reported Outcome: Negative

Myers looked at 374 children with cancer between 1970 and 1979, and 588 children who did not have cancer. All were less than sixteen years old. The study estimated exposures by determining the proximity of each participant's home to nearby power lines and calculating field levels based on the peak recorded load on the lines during the year in which the participant was born. This method is considered somewhat unreliable since it does not account for field levels within homes or variations over time. Myers reported no statistically significant associations between childhood cancer and either calculated field levels or, more simply, distance from power lines.

Myers, A, Clayden, AD, et al. (1990). "Childhood Cancer and Overhead Power Lines: A Case-Control Study." British Journal of Cancer *62: 1009–1014.*

Study authors: Ahlbom and Feychting
Date Published: 1993
Study type: Case-control
Reported Outcome: Positive

This study, in combination with an occupational EM field exposure study (Floderus 1993) and the other studies completed since 1979, led the Swedish government to announce in September 1992 that it would "act on the assumption that there is a connection between exposure to power frequency magnetic fields and cancer, in particular childhood cancer."

Ahlbom and Feychting evaluated everyone in Sweden who lived within 300 meters (about 980 feet) of either a 220 kilovolt or a 400 kilovolt transmission line in Sweden from 1960 through 1985—more than 400,000 people. Exposures were calculated using historical data on the amount of current on the line. In addition, the researchers took spot readings that were correlated to calculated fields (also based on current loads). The study considered adult leukemia and brain tumors, as well as all childhood cancers. (See page 176 for the results for adults.)

The investigators found an association between exposures and childhood leukemia, but not between EM fields and other childhood cancers. The leukemia risk increased proportionally along with the exposure level, indicative of what is known as a dose-response relationship. At 2 milligauss and above, exposed children were 2.7 times as likely to develop cancer as unexposed children, and at 3 milligauss and above the odds rose to 3.8 times as likely. These results were statistically significant; the researchers tried but could not explain the findings as a result of other factors. They also reported a slight association with distance from the transmission lines, but no association with spot measurements.

The researchers believe that their results help to explain why prior studies had found associations between wire coding and childhood cancer but not between measurements and childhood cancer. In a summary of their research released by the Swedish government, they explained:

> The finding of an association, in childhood leukemia, with calculated historical fields but not with measurements is consistent with the assumption that historical calculated fields are reasonably good predictors of past fields but that spot measurements are poor predictors of those fields.

Ahlbom, A and Feychting, M (1993). "Magnetic Fields and Cancer in Children Residing Near Swedish High Voltage Power Lines." American Journal of Epidemiology *138, no. 7: 467–481.*

Brain and Nervous System Cancers Among Children of Parents in Electrical Occupations

Researchers have done seven studies that evaluate the occupations of parents as a possible risk factor for brain cancers and cancers of the central nervous system (eg., the optic nerve). The underlying assumption is that exposure to EM fields might cause genetic damage that could lead to cancer in children.

Of the following studies, four relied on birth certificates for information about birth characteristics (weight, parental age, etc.) and about parental occupations. This method is not always reliable. The balance of the studies used telephone interviews to obtain the data. Interviews are often more reliable than birth certificates, though this method, too, can bias the study.

Study authors: Spitz and Johnson
Date Published: 1985
Study type: Case-control
Reported Outcome: Positive

The researchers analyzed the father's occupation for possible links to central nervous system cancer. They studied 157 deaths due to neuroblastomas of children less than fifteen years old. Neuroblastomas are nervous system cancers. The cases were matched with 314 controls. Birth certificates were the source of the father's occupation, with job title serving as a surrogate for EM field exposures. No measurements were made.

The study found that children of fathers who worked in EM field occupations were at a statistically significant increased risk of developing a neuroblastoma. One group of workers among the EM field occupations—electronic workers—was at a particularly high risk.

Spitz, MR and Johnson, CC (1985). "Neuroblastoma and Paternal Occupation: A Case-control Analysis." American Journal of Epidemiology *121: 924–929.*

Study authors: Wilkins and Koutras
Date Published: 1988
Study type: Case-control
Reported Outcome: Positive

This study evaluated 491 children who died of brain cancer between 1959 and 1978 in Ohio and 491 controls. All of the children in the study were Caucasian, less than twenty years old, and born before 1968. The father's occupation was taken from the birth certificate. The researchers reported a significantly increased risk of nearly three times for children whose fathers worked in electrical assembling, electrical installations, and electrical repair.

Wilkins, JR and Koutras, RA (1988). "Paternal Occupation and Brain Cancer in Offspring—A Mortality-based Case-control Study." American Journal of Industrial Medicine *14: 299–318.*

Study authors: Johnson and Spitz
Date Published: 1989
Study type: Case-control
Reported Outcome: Positive

Johnson and Spitz studied 499 children under fifteen years who had died with nervous system tumors between 1964 and 1980. They matched the cases with 998 controls and used birth certificate data to determine parental occupations. Children of construction electricians were at high risk of developing nervous system tumors, and children of all electricians were at low risk. Both findings were statistically significant.

Johnson, CC and Spitz, MR (1989). "Childhood Nervous System Tumors: An Assessment of Risk Associated with Paternal Occupations Involving Use, Repair, or Manufacture of Electrical and Electronic Equipment." International Journal of Epidemiology *18: 756–762.*

Study authors: Wilkins and Hundley
Date Published: 1990
Study type: Case-control
Reported Outcome: Negative

Wilkins and Hundley examined 101 children with neuroblastomas and 404 children as controls. All of the cases occurred from 1942 to 1967 in Columbus, Ohio. Parental occupation data came from birth certificates. They also evaluated the potential role of a wide range of factors including birth weight, prematurity, and the age of the parents at birth.

They found an increased risk associated with work in EM field occupations but it was not statistically significant.

Wilkins, JR and Hundley, VD (1990). "Paternal Occupational Exposure to Electromagnetic Fields and Neuroblastoma in Offspring." American Journal of Epidemiology *131, no. 6: 995–1008.*

Study author: Nasca
Date Published: 1988
Study type: Case-control
Reported Outcome: Negative

This study included 338 children less than fifteen years old who were diagnosed with nervous system tumors from 1968 through 1977. The controls totaled 676 children. Parents provided the data about diagnoses and parental occupations during telephone interviews with the research team. Exposure was estimated based on occupations. The study found no significant link with either the father's or the mother's presumed EM field exposures.

Nasca, PC, et al. (1988). "An Epidemiologic Case-control Study of Central Nervous System Tumors in Children and Parental Occupational Exposure." American Journal of Epidemiology *128: 1256–1265.*

Study author: Bunin
Date Published: 1990
Study type: Case-control
Reported Outcome: Negative

A study of 104 children diagnosed with neuroblastomas between 1970 and 1979 and an equal number of controls in metropolitan Philadelphia, Pennsylvania, did not find a significant association with the father's occupation prior to conception. The researchers gathered data via telephone interviews.

Bunin, GR, Ward, E, Kramer, S, et al. (1990). "Neuro-blastoma and Parental Occupation." American Journal of Epidemiology *131: 776–780.*

Study author: Kuijten
Date Published: 1992
Study type: Case-control
Reported Outcome: Positive

Kuijten's team evaluated 163 children with astrocytomas (a type of brain tumor) and 163 controls, all less than fifteen years of age and living in one of three Mid-Atlantic states. All of the cancers were diagnosed from 1980 to 1986. Using telephone interviews, the researchers obtained work histories for both parents. The study found that children whose fathers worked as electrical repairmen with presumed EM field exposures prior to conception were eight times as likely to have developed astrocytomas. This finding was statistically significant.

Kuijten, RR, Bunin, GR, Nass, CC, Meadows, AT (1992). "Parental Occupation and Childhood Astrocytoma: Results of a Case-control Study." Cancer Research *52: 782–786.*

Adult Cancer

Epidemiological research exploring the possible link between EM field exposures and cancers among adults is more extensive and more ambiguous than the work on childhood cancers. The majority of research involves workers, and these are known as occupational studies (see following section).

Residential studies are done for several reasons. First, some researchers wanted to assess the usefulness and validity of the methods used in the childhood cancer studies. Second, high EM field exposures from electric blankets could only be studied in homes. Third, investigators want to know whether the risks associated with EM fields are due to exposures from external sources (eg., transmission and distribution lines) or from internal sources (eg., house wiring, appliances).

Study authors: Wertheimer and Leeper
Date Published: 1982
Study type: Case-control
Reported Outcome: Positive

Wertheimer and Leeper used the wire code method they had developed earlier (see 1979 study, pages 160–162) to evaluate whether adults living near electrical wires faced a higher risk of dying from cancer than other adults.

They identified the homes of 1,179 cancer cases and matched them with an equal number of locations where people had died of causes other than cancer. Both groups were selected from several Colorado cities and included deaths from 1967 to 1975.

As they did in their 1979 study of childhood cancers, they found a statistically significant association between wire codes and cancer. They did not report any measurements. The researchers also concluded that the data suggested a dose-response relationship (the risk increased proportionally as the exposure levels increased) between wire codes and adult cancers, which would strengthen the case for an association.

Wertheimer, N and Leeper, E (1982). "Adult Cancer Related to Electrical Wires Near the Home." International Journal of Epidemiology *11: 345–355.*

Study author: McDowall
Date Published: 1986
Study type: Cohort
Reported Outcome: Negative

This negative study examined the causes of death for 7,631 people who lived near transmission lines in one community in 1971. McDowall examined cancer deaths among the population from 1971 to 1983.

The study found a statistically significant increase in lung cancer deaths among women and a significant increase in lung cancer among all people living within fourteen meters (about forty-six feet) of a line. Because the study did not collect data on smoking, however, these results are virtually impossible to interpret. Other cancers, including leukemia, brain cancer, and all cancers combined, did not occur at a higher than expected rate during the study period.

McDowall, ME (1986). "Mortality of Persons Resident in the Vicinity of Electricity Transmission Facilities." British Journal of Cancer *53: 271–279.*

Study authors: Wertheimer and Leeper
Date Published: 1987
Study type: Case-control
Reported Outcome: Positive

Wertheimer and Leeper reanalyzed the data from their 1982 study to look at specific cancer types. The methodology is the same as that analysis (see page 172). The investigators found significantly increased rates for cancers of the central nervous system, the reproductive system (all organs) and the uterus (separately), and the breast.

Wertheimer, N and Leeper, E (1987). "Magnetic Field Exposure Related to Cancer Subtypes." Annals of the New York Academy of Sciences *502: 43–54.*

Study author: Preston-Martin
Date Published: 1988
Study type: Case-control
Reported Outcome: Negative

Unlike most of the studies discussed so far, this one looked at two specific type of cancer—acute and chronic myelogenous (also called myelocytic) leukemias—and one specific type of exposure—electric blanket use. As with all leukemias, acute myelogenous leukemia and chronic myelogenous leukemia involve uncontrolled and destructive growth of abnormal, immature white blood cells. Both types commonly occur in people of all ages. Electric blankets expose people to fairly high EM field levels—as high as 300 milligauss within one-half inch of the blanket—and are presumed to be a predictable exposure source for studies. That is, if people use electric blankets, you can for the sake of study assume that they are exposed to high fields for six to eight hours on most days during cold seasons.

Preston-Martin identified 116 cases of acute myelogenous leukemia and 108 cases of chronic myelogenous leukemia as well as 228 controls in Los Angeles County, California, between mid-1979 and mid-1985. They found no statistically significant association between either type of cancer and electric blanket use. Exposure was based on whether the participants said they used electric blankets regularly, and the investigators did not attempt to learn whether the participants who used electric blankets did so year-round, sporadically, or only on cold nights. The researchers recommended that a comparable study be tried in a colder climate.

Preston-Martin, S, Peters, JM, Yu, MC (1988). "Myelogenous Leukemia and Electric Blanket Use." Bioelectromagnetics *9: 207–213.*

Study author: Severson
Date Published: 1988
Study type: Case-control
Reported Outcome: Negative

One of many studies to include both wire coding–based exposure estimates and a limited number of spot measurements, this investigation included 114 people with acute nonlymphocytic leukemia and 133 controls, all living in the western part of Washington state. The researchers also used a questionnaire to estimate exposures from appliances; when people had died, the next-of-kin answered the questionnaires. The study found no significant associations for wire codes or spot measurements.

Severson, RK, Stevens, RG, Kaune, WT, et al. (1988). "Acute Nonlymphocytic Leukemia and Residential Exposure to Power Frequency Magnetic Fields." American Journal of Epidemiology *128: 10–20.*

Study author: Coleman
Date Published: 1989
Study type: Case-control
Reported Outcome: Negative

Coleman and his colleagues used a surrogate other than wire codes to estimate EM field exposures at homes near transmission lines and substations. For transmission lines, they measured the distances from the lines to the homes. For substations, they developed an exposure index that calculated field strength based on the peak electricity demand during the winter, adjusted for the rate at which the field strength decreases over distance.

The investigators selected 771 people diagnosed with leukemia from 1965 through 1980; 1,432 cancer controls (people with cancer who did not live near transmission lines or substations); and 231 controls from the general population. This included 84 children with cancer and 141 children in the control group.

The data included some interesting, though nonsignificant, findings. Children under eighteen years who lived within 50 meters (about 164 feet) of a substation had a 50 percent increased risk of leukemia; anyone living within 50 meters of a transmission line had a 100 percent increased risk of leukemia; anyone living within 100 meters of a line had a 45 percent increased risk; and anyone within 25 meters of a substation had a 30 percent increased risk of leukemia.

Coleman, MP, Bell, CMJ, et al. (1989). "Leukemia and Residence Near Electricity Transmission Equipment: A Case-Control Study." British Journal of Cancer *60: 793–798.*

Study authors: Ahlbom and Feychting
Date Published: 1993
Study type: Case-control
Reported Outcome: Negative

This study looked at both childhood cancers (see page 166) and adult cancers, particularly acute myeloid leukemia and chronic myeloid leukemia. It found 70 percent increases of both diseases for adults exposed to EM fields greater than 2 milligauss, but neither finding was statistically significant.

Ahlbom, A and Feychting, M (1993). "Magnetic Fields and Cancer in Children Residing Near Swedish High Voltage Power Lines." American Journal of Epidemiology *138, no. 7: 467-481.*

Study author: Schreiber
Date Published: 1993
Study type: Cohort
Reported Outcome: Negative

A team of Dutch researchers found no significant association between proximity to transmission lines or substations and any single type of cancer or all cancers combined. The study involved 431 deaths—192 of which involved people who lived for at least five years within 100 meters (about 328 feet) of either two transmission lines or a substation, and 239 of which involved people who did not. The researchers cautioned that the small number of cancer cases limited the statistical power of the study.

Schreiber, G, et al. (1993). "Cancer Mortality and Residence near Electricity Transmission Equipment: A Retrospective Cohort Study." International Journal of Epidemiology *22: 9–15.*

Adult Occupational Cancers

Generally, it is less difficult and less costly to identify a study population among groups of workers than it is among the general public. Workers' records are usually more detailed and more accessible, and their exposures often are more reliably obtained or calculated. In addition, confounding factors such as exposures to toxic chemicals are easier to document for groups of workers than for people at home.

Research has focused on three types of cancer: leukemia, brain cnacer, and male breast cancer. The latter two may prove particularly important to investigators because they are rare and therefore easier to study apart from confounding factors. Male breast cancer findings also have raised important questions about female breast cnacer.

Leukemia

Study author: Wiklund
Date Published: 1981
Study type: Standardized incidence ratio
Reported Outcome: Negative

Wiklund calculated on the basis of recorded cancer rates that you would expect to see 11.7 cases of leukemia among all of the telephone operators at the Swedish Telecommunications Administration in Goteborg from 1969 through 1974. By reviewing records of the workers he identified twelve cases, and the small difference was not significant.

Wiklund, K, Einhorn, J, and Eklund, G (1981). "An Application of the Swedish Cancer-Environment Registry. Leukemia Among Telephone Operators at the Telecommunications Administration in Sweden." International Journal of Epidemiology *10: 373–376.*

Study author: Milham
Date Published: 1982
Study type: Proportional mortality ratio
Reported Outcome: Positive

Milham's analysis, published as a letter rather than as a peer-reviewed paper, was the first to report a positive association between occupational EM field exposures and leukemia. By examining deaths from leukemia among white men in Washington state from 1950 to 1979 and by grouping the deaths according to the occupation listed on death certificates, Milham found several statistically significant cancer associations. Electricians, power station workers, and aluminum workers all had significant associations. In addition, all electrical occupations grouped together had significant associations for both all leukemias in general and for a specific type known as acute leukemia in particular.

Milham presumed EM field exposures based on his knowledge of various industries and his ability to distinguish jobs that involved prolonged proximity to higher-than-average field levels. Many other researchers have also estimated exposure by job category, and it is an accepted, if imprecise, epidemiological method. Milham and most other researchers who used this method have not taken measurements.

Milham, S, Jr (1982). "Mortality from Leukemia in Workers Exposed to Electrical and Magnetic Fields" (letter). New England Journal of Medicine *307: 249.*

Study author: Wright
Date Published: 1982
Study type: Proportional incidence ratio
Reported Outcome: Positive

In another letter to a respected, peer-reviewed scientific journal, Wright reported a statistically significant increase in the occurrence of acute leukemias among thirty-five white men working in electrical professions. He drew his cases from workers in Los Angeles County, California, between 1972 and 1979.

Wright also found that power linemen (who install and fix power transmission and distribution wires) were particularly at an increased risk: they were almost six times as likely to develop acute leukemia as men working in nonelectrical occupations. Like Milham, Wright used job occupation as a surrogate for exposures. No measurements were taken.

Wright, WE, Peters, JM, Mack, TM (1982). "Leukemia in Workers Exposed to Electrical and Magnetic Fields" (letter). Lancet *ii: 1160–1161. November 20, 1982.*

Study author: McDowall
Date Published: 1983
Study type: Proportional mortality ratio/case-control
Reported Outcomes: Negative (proportional mortality ratio) and positive (case-control)

In an evaluation of 98 leukemia deaths among men, McDowall found increased rates of leukemia for telegraph radio operators, but the finding was not significant. As Milham and Wright had done, McDowall used job titles as a surrogate for exposures. As a second phase of his study, McDowall also reported on a case-control study of 537 men who died of acute myeloid leukemia and 1,074 controls. Again he used job titles to estimate exposures, but this time he found a statistically significant increase—a near-doubling of risk—for men working in electrical occupations.

McDowall, ME (1983). "Leukemia Mortality in Electrical Workers in England and Wales" (letter). Lancet *i: 246. January 29, 1983.*

Study author: Coleman
Date Published: 1983
Study type: Proportional incidence ratio
Reported Outcome: Positive

Using the job title method of assessing exposure, this study found a statistically significant increase in the incidence of leukemia for some electrical workers, particularly telegraph-radio operators. The increase was highest for chronic myeloid leukemia among this group of workers. In general, though not all of the increases were significant, most of the ten occupations studied showed increased risk of leukemia.

Coleman, M, Bell J, and Skeet, R (1983). "Leukemia Incidence in Electrical Workers" (letter). Lancet *i: 982-983. April 30, 1983.*

Study author: Calle and Savitz
Date Published: 1985
Study type: Proportional mortality ratio
Reported Outcome: Negative

Calle and Savitz used the same methods as Milham (1982) and Wright (1982) but reported different results. They evaluated the occupations for eighty-one white men who died of leukemia between 1963 and 1978. In part, this research was designed to test the use of job titles as a surrogate for EM field exposures. On the basis of their findings, Calle and Savitz urged caution in further use of this method. Those conclusions notwithstanding, the study produced statistically significant associations between electrical occupations and some types of cancer. In particular, the study linked leukemia and electrical engineers and leukemia and radio-telegraph operators.

Calle, EE and Savitz, DA (1985). "Leukemia in Occupational Groups with Presumed Exposure to Electric and Magnetic Fields" (letter). New England Journal of Medicine *313: 1476–1477.*

Study author: Gilman
Date Published: 1985
Study type: Case-control
Reported Outcome: Positive

This study was limited by methodological shortcomings, not the least of which was its limited consideration of factors other than EM fields as potential leukemia-causing agents. Coal mines are notoriously hazardous environments.

Gilman compared 40 leukemia deaths among coal miners to 160 controls who died from a natural cause other than cancer. All study subjects were white males. Electrical wiring in coal mines is generally very close to the workers, and EM field exposure levels are presumed to be high. Gilman's team did not make measurements. The investigators found statistically significant increases for all leukemias (a 253 percent rise), chronic leukemia (an 800 percent rise), chronic lymphocytic leukemia (630 percent rise), and myelogenous leukemia (474 percent rise), all for men who had been working in the underground coal mines at least twenty-five years.

Gilman, PA, Ames, RG, McCawley, MA (1985). "Leukemia Risk Among US White Male Coal Miners." Journal of Occupational Medicine 27: 669–671.

Study author: Milham
Date Published: 1985
Study type: Proportional mortality ratio
Reported Outcome: Positive

Milham examined the death certificates of 1,691 ham radio operators and compared the causes of their deaths to those in the general population. All of the subjects died in either Washington state or California between 1971 and 1983.

The study found a statistically significant increase in cases of myeloid leukemia and in all leukemias combined but no significant increase in other specific types of leukemias. No measurements were taken, and exposure was assumed on the basis of membership in the American Radio Relay League, the ham radio association. Because ham radio operators work close to numerous electrical and electronic devices, their exposures are thought to be higher than average.

Milham, S, Jr (1985). "Silent Keys: Leukemia Mortality in Amateur Radio Operators" (letter). Lancet i: 812. April 6, 1985.

Study author: Pearce
Date Published: 1985, 1988
Study type: Case-control
Reported Outcome: Positive

Working with 564 cases of leukemia and 2,184 cases of other types of cancer, Pearce found that electricians were almost five times as likely and radio and television repairmen were more than eight times as likely to develop leukemia. The size of the study population gave it statistical power, and the use of leukemia and cancer incidence rather than mortality (i.e., taking information about participants' jobs at the time they developed cancer rather than at the time of their deaths, thereby linking the disease and the work more closely) added to the accuracy of the results. On the other hand, the study design did not attempt to weed out other possible leukemia-causing factors, or confounders, and the use of people with cancer types other than leukemia could be a problem if any or all of these cancer types are also associated to EM field exposures.

Pearce, NE, Sheppard, RA, Howard, JK, et al. (1985). "Leukemia in Electrical Workers in New Zealand" (letter). Lancet *i: 811–812.*

Pearce, NE (1988). "Leukemia in Electrical Workers in New Zealand: A Correction" (letter). Lancet: 48.

Study author: Flodin
Date Published: 1986
Study type: Case-control
Reported Outcome: Positive

Flodin compared occupational and personal data about 59 leukemia cases and 354 controls. EM field exposure was determined by job title. The study found a significant association between electrical workers and leukemia after adjusting the data to allow for possible confounders, including solvent exposure and smoking. The careful inclusion of these factors added to the study's strength.

Flodin, U, Fredricksson, M, Axelson, O, et al. (1986). "Background Radiation, Electrical Work, and Some Other Exposures Associated with Acute Myeloid Leukemia in a Case-Referent Study." Archives of Environmental Health *411: 77–84.*

Study author: Stern
Date Published: 1986
Study type: Case-control
Reported Outcome: Positive

This investigation looked at 53 leukemia deaths and 212 controls at a U.S. Navy facility in Portsmouth, New Hampshire. Instead of using death certificates to determine job titles, the researchers used military duty records, which gave the study more precision. They also used the duty records to estimate duration of work and, hence, exposure. All of the deaths occurred from 1952 through 1981. Stern found that electricians were three times as likely to have died of leukemia. Electrical shop personnel were slightly less likely. Both figures were statistically significant.

Stern, FB, Waxweiler, RA, Beaumont, JJ, et al. (1986). "A Case-Control Study of Leukemia at a Naval Nuclear Shipyard." American Journal of Epidemiology *123:980–992.*

Study author: Linet
Date Published: 1988
Study type: Standardized incidence ratio
Reported Outcome: Positive

In this study, Linet evaluated 5,351 leukemia cases

between 1961 and 1979 in terms of their job classifications. She evaluated the data for all leukemias and also for specific types of leukemia. She found no significant increase among all electrical workers as a group, but she did observe that power line workers experienced nearly double the risk as nonelectrical workers of developing chronic lymphocytic leukemia. This finding was statistically significant.

Linet, MS (1988). "Leukemias and Occupation in Sweden—A Registry-based Analysis." American Journal of Industrial Medicine 14: 319–330.

Study authors: Preston-Martin and Peters
Date Published: 1988
Study type: Case-control
Reported Outcome: Positive

Electric arc welding is known to produce notably high EM field levels. This study was part of a large study of leukemia in Los Angeles County, California. So high was the incidence of chronic myeloid leukemia among welders— twenty-five times as high as nonwelders—that the researchers published the arc welders' data separate from the broader leukemia results.

Using 130 people who had developed leukemia and 130 who had not, Preston-Martin and Peters identified 22 cases and 4 controls who had worked as welders at some time. After factoring in other possible leukemia-causing agents, the researchers found that welding is associated with at least one type of cancer. They did not attempt to make EM field measurements or estimate exposures from metal fumes, however.

Preston-Martin S and Peters, J (1988). "Prior Employment as a Welder Associated with the Development of Chronic Myeloid Leukemia" (note). British Journal of Cancer 58: 105–108.

Study author: Bastuji-Garin
Date Published: 1990
Study type: Case-control
Reported Outcome: Positive

This French research team used data from interviews of 185 people with acute myelogenous leukemia and 513 others serving as controls to evaluate the role of EM field exposures, solvent exposures, and other factors. After adjusting for possible confounding factors, the researchers found a statistically significant association between EM field exposures and acute myelogenous leukemia. The use of estimated exposures based on interviews made this study stronger than those using job titles.

Bastuji-Garin, S, Richardson, S, and Zittoun, R (1990). "Acute Leukemia in Workers Exposed to Electromagnetic Fields." European Journal of Cancer *26: 1119–1120.*

Study author: Gallagher
Date Published: 1990
Study type: Proportional mortality ratio
Reported Outcome: Negative

Using job titles taken from death certificates, Gallagher evaluated sixty-five leukemia deaths that occurred between 1950 and 1984 in British Columbia, Canada. He found no significant association between leukemia and electrical and electronic assemblers and repairmen aged twenty to sixty-five years.

Gallagher, RP, McBride, ML, et al. (1990). "Occupational Electromagnetic Field Exposure, Solvent Exposure, and Leukemia" (letter). Journal of Occupational Medicine *32: 64–65.*

Study author: Garland
Date Published: 1990
Study type: Standardized incidence ratio
Reported Outcome: Positive

Among 102 cases of leukemia drawn from U.S. Navy personnel worldwide, Garland's team identified one electrical occupation—electrician's mate—that had a statistically significant association to leukemia. The increased risk was almost two-and-a-half times the expected rate, but the number of cases (seven) was small, making the finding less reliable than it would have been if the number of cases was much larger.

Garland, FC, Shaw, E, Gorham, ED, et al. (1990). "Incidence of Leukemia in Occupations with Potential Electromagnetic field Exposure in United States Navy Personnel." American Journal of Epidemiology *132: 293–303.*

Study author: Robinson
Date Published: 1991
Study type: Proportional mortality ratio
Reported Outcome: Positive

This study included 183 deaths from leukemia among white men in fourteen states, using job titles taken from death certificates. The study population was selected from more than 425,000 deaths.

Robinson found a statistically significant increase for all leukemias among electrical workers, and another significant increase in acute myelogenous leukemia among telephone-telegraph operators and other communications equipment users. Telephone linemen and repairmen had nearly a 250 percent increase in acute myelogenous leukemia risk but it was not statistically significant. Robinson, who was with the National Institute for Occupational Safety and Health, reported that her team's findings confirmed prior results showing that "occupational exposure in electrical occupations may be associated with enhanced leukemia risk."

Robinson, CF, Sesito, JP, and Fine, LJ (1991). "Electromagnetic Field Exposure and Leukemia Mortality in the United States." Journal of Occupational Medicine 33: 160—162.

Study author: Richardson
Date Published: 1992
Study type: Case-control
Reported Outcome: Positive

This investigation comprised 185 people over thirty years of age with acute leukemia in two Paris hospitals and 513 controls. The controls were hospital patients matched to the cases on the basis of gender, age, ethnic group, and residence, though they did not necessarily represent the general population. The investigators interviewed all the participants about their work histories and related information. They developed a method for assigning an EM field "dose" rating to each participant on the basis of the interviews. For their analysis, the researchers excluded both cases and controls who were electric arc welders, who are exposed to a range of metal and chemical fumes. The resulting data showed a statistically significant increase in acute myelogenous leukemias among the EM exposed population, although the study did not find an association with either EM field levels or exposure duration. Richardson's team concluded that the study "adds credence" to the hypothesis that EM fields are associated with cancer. That hypothesis, they wrote, "has reached consistency." The team that did this study also did the study identified above as Bastuji-Garin (1990).

Richardson, S, Zittoun, R, Bastuji-Garin, S, et al. (1992). "Occupational Risk Factors for Acute Leukemia: A Case-Con-

trol Study." International Journal of Epidemiology *21: 1063–1073.*

Study author: Matanoski
Date Published: 1993
Study type: Case-control
Reported Outcome: Positive

This study was part of a larger project that also reported important findings for male breast cancer (Matanoski, 1991; see page 195). The larger project attracted a great deal of scientific, media, and public attention because Matanoski is widely regarded as one of the world's top epidemiologists. In 1993, the Environmental Protection Agency chose her to head its Science Advisory Board, a panel of experts responsible for reviewing the agency's major scientific research, analyses, and research plans.

The study also is one of the most thorough completed to date. Matanoski identified 124 workers with leukemia and 372 controls. All study participants worked for AT&T, the telecommunications company. For 75 of the cases and 196 of the controls, the researchers simply worked with job titles. But for 35 cases and 77 controls, the researchers developed complete work histories. For each participant, they calculated an exposure "score" based on EM field measurements they took and the duration of the jobs performed. The study found a statistically significant link between cancer risk and increasing exposure levels, a dose-response relationship. At the same time, however, they found that none of the groups of workers they studied individually had a significantly increased risk.

Matanoski, GM, Elliott, EA, et al. (1993). "Leukemia in Telephone Linemen." American Journal of Epidemiology *137: 609–619.*

Study author: Thériault
Date Published: 1994
Study type: Case-control
Reported Outcome: Positive

In a study of 4,151 cancer cases between 1970 and 1989 among workers at three electric power utilities in Canada and France, Thériault's team found statistically significant increased risks for two types of leukemia (acute nonlymphoid leukemia and acute myeloid leukemia). The researchers did not observe a dose-response relationship— that is, the risk did not increase proportionate to increasing exposure levels. The study also found a trend of increased brain cancer risk among the workers, but the finding was not statistically significant. They found no association between exposure and male breast cancer, prostate cancer, or any of twenty-seven other types of cancer.

The study size—more than 220,000 men were involved—and the exposure assessment method made this a strong study. The investigators measured exposures of more than 2,000 workers doing jobs similar to those in the study and also calculated past exposures. The authors note that the study does not provide conclusive evidence of an EM field-cancer link. The primary difficulty they identified was in reaching accurate exposure data. "It remains possible that our observation was due to chance, but it is more likely that the inconsistencies in our results correspond to the as yet underestimated difficulty of arriving at an accurate exposure estimate for each study participant," they wrote.

Thériault, G, Goldberg, M, et al. (1994). "Cancer Risks Associated with Occupational Exposure to Magnetic Fields among Electric Utility Workers in Ontario and Quebec, Canada, and France: 1970-1989." American Journal of Epidemiology *138: 550–572.*

Brain Cancer

Study author: Preston-Martin
Date Published: 1982
Study type: Proportional incidence ratio
Reported Outcome: Positive

Preston-Martin identified 1,529 men and 1,686 women with brain tumors in Los Angeles County, California, for the years 1972–1977. Using job titles listed on cancer registry forms, her team found significantly increased rates of brain cancer among electricians and among engineers.

Preston-Martin, S, Henderson, BE, and Peters, JM (1982). "Descriptive Epidemiology of Central Nervous System Neoplasms in Los Angeles County." Annals of the New York Academy of Sciences *381: 202–208.*

Study author: Lin
Date Published: 1985
Study type: Proportional mortality ratio, case-control
Reported Outcome: Positive

This study was done in two parts. The proportional mortality analysis found a significant excess of two types of primary brain cancers—gliomas and astrocytomas. Primary brain cancers are those that originate in the brain as opposed to those that spread to the brain after originating elsewhere. The case-control analysis involved 951 white men who died of brain cancer between 1969 and 1982, and 951 men serving as controls. Lin found that men who had worked in electrical occupations had died of brain cancer at a significantly higher rate than men who did not.

Lin, RS, Dischinger, PC, Conde, J, et al. (1985). "Occupational Exposure to Electromagnetic Fields and the Occurrence of Brain Tumors." Journal of Occupational Medicine *27: 413–419.*

Study author: McLaughlin
Date Published: 1987
Study type: Standardized incidence ratio
Reported Outcome: Negative

Based on a study of 3,394 cases of brain tumors in Swedish men from 1961 through 1979, McLaughlin found no significant risk associated with working in electrical occupations. Exposure was presumed on the basis of job titles in the 1960 Swedish census.

McLaughlin, JK, Malker, HSR, Blot, WJ, et al. (1987). "Occupational Risks for Intracranial Gliomas in Sweden." Journal of the National Cancer Institute *78: 253–257.*

Study author: Thomas
Date Published: 1987
Study type: Case-control
Reported Outcome: Positive

Using 435 brain tumor cases and 386 controls, this study relied on interviews with survivors to establish work history, job title(s), exposure to power frequency EM fields, exposure to EM radiation, and exposure to other agents. This method of data collection is considered better than job titles from death certificates but not as good as information from personnel records. The study found a significantly increased risk of astrocytomas—a type of brain tumor—among workers in electronics manufacturing and repair jobs. Equally important, the data showed a statistically significant trend of increased risk with increased years of exposure.

Thomas, TL, Stolley, PD, et al. (1987). "Brain Tumor Mortality Risk Among Men with Electrical and Electronics Jobs: A Case-control Study." Journal of the National Cancer Institute *79: 233–238.*

Study author: Speers
Date Published: 1988
Study type: Case-control
Reported Outcome: Positive

Matching 200 people who died from gliomas—a type of primary brain cancer—to 238 controls, this study based exposure estimates on job titles taken from death certificates. All deaths occurred from 1969 to 1978. Utility workers, electricians, electronics workers, and others believed to have been exposed to EM fields were significantly more likely to develop gliomas.

Speers, MA, Dobbins, JG, Miller, VS (1988). "Occupational Exposures and Brain Cancer Mortality: A Preliminary Study of East Texas Residents." American Journal of Industrial Medicine *13: 629–638.*

Study author: Mack
Date Published: 1991
Study type: Case-control
Reported Outcome: Positive

This strong study included 272 adult men with brain cancer and the same number of controls. The researchers interviewed the participants in the period 1980–1984, gathering extensive information including complete job histories with the duration of each job done. Getting this data from the participants directly rather than through interviews with family members or from death certificates is a major strength of this study.

The investigation produced two statistically significant results. First, men who had worked for at least ten years in an electrical occupation were much more likely to have developed an astrocytoma (a primary brain cancer) than were the controls. Second, the longer a participant worked the more likely he was to develop brain cancer, a possible dose-response relationship.

Mack, W, Preston-Martin, S, Peters, J (1991). "Astrocytoma Risk Related to Job Exposure to Electric and Magnetic Fields." Bioelectromagnetics *12: 57–66.*

Male Breast Cancer

Male breast cancer is a very rare disease. Most epidemiologists and public health officials consider the series of positive findings for male breast cancer very important, for two reasons. First, its rarity makes an excess notable and more easily studied than other types of cancer that are known to result from several different factors. Second, male breast cancer and female breast cancer are similar. Because there is an epidemic of female breast cancer in the United States (approximately one woman in nine will develop breast cancer in her lifetime), the male breast cancer findings may help scientists identify a cause of the female breast cancer epidemic.

Study author: Tynes
Date Published: 1990
Study type: Standardized incidence ratio
Reported Outcome: Positive

Tynes found a significant link between male breast cancer and work in all electrical occupations, and particularly work in electrical transport jobs. He found 12 cases among almost 38,000 men working in Norway from 1961 to 1985, compared to the 5.8 cases predicted on the basis of historical cancer data. He derived job titles as surrogates for exposures from the 1960 and 1970 national censuses, and used the 1960 census to predict the expected number of cases.

Tynes, T and Andersen, A (1990). "Electromagnetic Fields and Male Breast Cancer" (letter). Lancet *336: 1596.*

Study author: Matanoski
Date Published: 1991
Study type: Standardized incidence ratio
Reported Outcome: Positive

As part of her large study of leukemia among telephone workers (Matanoski, 1993; see page 189), Matanoski identified two cases of male breast cancer, which is more than six times the number predicted by standardized cancer data. This finding was not statistically significant. Of note, Matanoski chose to exclude four additional cases of male breast cancer for technical reasons. She studied more than 50,000 telephone company employees, including more than 9,500 technicians many of whom worked near switching equipment known to emit fields of about 2.5 milligauss. All of the workers studied were employed by AT&T between 1976 and 1980.

Matanoski, BM, Breysse, PN, and Elliott, EA (1991). "Electromagnetic Field Exposure and Male Breast Cancer" (letter). Lancet *337:737.*

Study author: Demers
Date Published: 1991
Study type: Case-control
Reported Outcome: Positive

This strong study matched 227 men with breast cancer to 300 men without breast cancers as controls and found that electricians, telephone linemen, and electric power workers were six times as likely to develop breast cancer. Demers's team found that the risk was greatest for men first employed in those occupations (and presumably exposed) before age thirty and who had worked at least thirty years on the job. Both findings were statistically significant.

Using a classification scheme developed by another researcher, Demers found that men with "possible" EM field exposures were not more likely to develop breast cancer than unexposed men, men with "probable" exposures were slightly more likely, and men with "definite" exposures were much more likely. This, too, was a significant finding. Demers's team used personal interviews to collect information about job titles and working conditions.

Demers, PA, Thomas, DB, Rosenblatt, KA, et al. (1991). "Occupational Exposure to Electromagnetic Fields and Breast Cancer in Men." American Journal of Epidemiology *134: 340–347.*

Study author: Loomis
Date Published: 1992
Study type: Case-control
Reported Outcome: Negative

Loomis studied 250 men who died from breast cancer in the period 1985–1988 in comparison to 2,500 controls. He obtained job titles and related occupational information from death certificates. The investigation found four cases of breast cancer among the 250 cases. This was not a statistically significant increase.

Loomis, DP (1992). "Cancer of Breast Among Men in Electrical Occupations." Lancet *339: 1482–1483.*

Other Cancer Types

Study author: Guralnick
Date Published: 1963
Study type: Standardized mortality ratio
Reported Outcome: Positive

Guralnick evaluated 327,271 deaths that occurred in 1950, using job titles from death certificates. He found a significant excess for all cancers in stationary engineers, who were presumed to have higher-than-normal EM field exposures. Wertheimer and Leeper (1979) cited this study as one of the reasons for looking at EM field exposures in their landmark study.

Guralnick, L (1963). "Mortality by Occupation and Cause of Death Among Men 20 to 64 Years of Age, United States, 1950." U.S. Vital Statistics Special Reports 53.

Study authors: Vagero and Olin
Date Published: 1983
Study type: Cohort
Reported Outcome: Positive

The researchers studied 54,624 men and 18,478 women who in 1960 worked in the Swedish electronics industry. They obtained cancer rates from the Swedish national cancer registry for the period 1961–1973. For the men, they found significant associations with all cancer types and with numerous individual types. For women, they found associations with all cancer types and with uterine cancer. These findings were statistically significant.

Vagero, D and Olin, R (1983). "Incidence of Cancer in the Electronics Industry: Using the New Swedish Cancer Environmental Registry as a Screening Instrument." British Journal of Industrial Medicine 40: 188–192.

Study author: Milham
Date Published: 1985
Study type: Proportional mortality ratio
Reported Outcome: Positive

Studying 486,000 white men who died in Washington state between 1950 and 1982, Milham reported several statistically significant findings. For men in jobs with presumed EM field exposures, he found links to all malignant tumors, to all lymph-related and blood-related cancers, to all types of leukemia, and to acute leukemia. The study's size is a major strength, improving the probability that the findings are accurate. On the other hand, the use of job titles as a surrogate for exposure is a weakness.

Milham, S, Jr (1985). "Mortality in Workers Exposed to Electromagnetic Fields." Environmental Health Perspectives *62: 297–300.*

Study author: Tornqvist
Date Published: 1986
Study type: Standardized mortality ratio
Reported Outcome: Positive

For the period 1961–1979, 3,358 power linemen and 6,703 power station operators were studied for cancer incidence. The researchers obtained job titles from census data and used it as a surrogate for EM field exposures. Power linemen, who install and maintain power transmission lines, had a slightly increased risk of developing cancer, while power station operators had marginally increased rates of cancer of the urinary organs, including the kidneys. These results were statistically significant.

Tornqvist's team are among the premier epidemiologists in the field. Ahlbom's 1993 study was one of the studies that persuaded the Swedish government to adopt a policy based on the assumption that EM fields are linked to cancer.

Tornqvist, S, Norell, S, Ahlbom, A, Knave, B (1986). "Cancer in the Electric Power Industry." British Journal of Industrial Medicine *43: 212–213.*

Study authors: Wertheimer and Leeper
Date Published: 1987
Study type: Standardized mortality ratio, and
 Proportional mortality ratio
Reported Outcome: Positive

Wertheimer and Leeper reanalyzed the Guralnick (1963) data and the Milham (1985) data using job titles as surrogates for exposures. They found statistically significant increases for several types of cancer—lung, urinary, and nervous system.

Wertheimer, N and Leeper, E (1987). "Magnetic Field Exposure Related to Cancer Subtypes." Annals of the New York Academy of Sciences *502: 43–54.*

Study author: Milham
Date Published: 1988
Study type: Standardized mortality ratio
Reported Outcome: Negative

Unlike Milham's earlier studies (1982, 1985), this one did not find a statistically significant increase in cancer rates among men with presumed EM field exposures. In this investigation, Milham studied 67,829 amateur radio operator licensees in Washington and California who died between 1979 and 1984. He found a statistically significant *decrease* in all tumors and in pancreatic cancer deaths, but he also observed a marginally significant excess in lymph system and blood system cancers, as well as in acute myeloid leukemia, a disease that numerous other studies also have associated with exposure.

In a followup analysis, Milham considered the data according to the length of time the licensees had operated amateur radio systems and during which the operator presumably was exposed to EM fields. Among men with only modest exposures, Milham found the most striking results: increased risks for lymph and blood system cancers, multiple myelomas, and other lymphomas. These findings may reflect the presence of exposure "windows"—effects that occur under some, but not all, conditions. Laboratory research has found several such windows.

Milham, S, Jr (1988). "Increased Mortality in Amateur Radio Operators Due to Lymphatic and Hematopoietic Malignancies." American Journal of Epidemiology *127: 50–54.*

Milham, S, Jr (1988). "Mortality by License Class in Amateur Radio Operators." American Journal of Epidemiology *128: 1175–1176.*

Study author: Pearce
Date Published: 1989
Study type: Case-control
Reported Outcome: Positive

This study looked at the incidence of cancer among men working in electrical occupations in New Zealand. The cancer cases were all diagnosed between 1980 and 1984. Radio and television repairmen, power station operators, and power linemen all had significantly elevated leukemia rates in decreasing order.

Pearce, N, Reif, J, and Fraser, J (1989). "Case-control Studies of Cancer in New Zealand Electrical Workers." International Journal of Epidemiology *18: 55–59.*

Study author: Juutilainen
Date Published: 1990
Study type: Cohort
Reported Outcome: Positive

Juutilainen did a comprehensive study of all men working in Finland in 1970 and searched for cancer occurrences among them from 1971 through 1980. Using the 1970 census to obtain job titles, he classified the men according to probable and possible exposure classifications. Leukemia was associated with probable exposures, and the link was significant but marginal. Central nervous system cancer was associated with possible exposure, again significantly but marginally.

Juutilainen, J, Laara, E, Pukkala, E (1990). "Incidence of Leukemia and Brain Tumors in Finnish Workers Exposed to ELF Magnetic Fields." International Archives of Occupational and Environmental Health 62: 289—293.

Study authors: Loomis and Savitz
Date Published: 1990
Study type: Case-control
Reported Outcome: Positive (for brain cancer)

This strong study focused specifically on brain cancer and leukemia among electrical workers. All of the data, including job title, were derived from death certificates filed in 1985 and 1986 in sixteen states. Looking at brain cancer, the researchers matched 2,173 deaths to 21,730 deaths due to causes other than brain cancer or leukemia. They found that electrical workers in general had elevated risks, as did electrical and electronics engineers and technicians, telephone and telephone line installers and repair workers, and electric power equipment installers and repairers. These associations all were statistically significant. They also matched 3,400 leukemia deaths to 34,000 controls. There was no significant increase in risk.

Loomis, DP, and Savitz, DA (1990). "Brain Cancer and Leukemia Mortality Among Electrical Workers." British Journal of Industrial Medicine *47: 633–638.*

Study author: Tornqvist
Date Published: 1991
Study type: Standardized morbidity ratio
Reported Outcome: Positive

In a study of 133,687 men working in electrical occupations in Sweden, the Tornqvist team found statistically significant increases in leukemia for electronics engineers and for telegraph and telephone technicians. It also found a significant excess among radio–TV assemblers and repairmen for glioblastomas, a type of brain cancer. Exposures were assessed on the basis of job titles taken from the 1960 census, and the researchers used only those cancers diagnosed between 1961 and 1979.

Tornqvist, S, et al. (1991). "Incidence of Leukemia and Brain Tumors in Some Electrical Occupations." British Journal of Industrial Medicine *48: 597–603.*

Study author: Floderus
Date Published: 1993
Study type: Case-control
Reported Outcome: Positive

Floderus's study was the second of two studies that led the Swedish government to develop a policy predicated on the assumption that EM field exposures are associated with cancer (see also Ahlbom and Feychting, 1993). A second outstanding characteristic of the Floderus investigation is the finding that cancer risk rose as exposures increased, suggesting a dose–response relationship.

The study matched 250 men with leukemia and 261 men with brain tumors to 1,121 controls. Floderus measured field levels, taking some 25 million readings involving 169 job categories. She classified the study participants in four categories, according to their mean daily exposures. Those workers in the top quarter were significantly more likely to have developed leukemia in general and chronic lymphocytic leukemia in particular. There was no significant association between exposures and acute lymphocytic leukemia. The data strongly suggested that the leukemia link was not related to other agents such as ionizing radiation, pesticides, solvents, and smoking.

The study found suggestions of a dose–response association between EM field exposures and brain cancer, but the link was weaker than it was for leukemia. Floderus concluded that several factors—such as the age of workers when they are first exposed on the job, workers' cumulative exposures, and age at diagnosis—need further study. Overall, Floderus found, "The results of this study speak in favor of the hypothesis that occupational EM field exposure is a hazard in the development of certain cancers."

Floderus, B (1992). "Occupational Exposure to Electromagnetic Fields in Relation to Leukemia and Brain Tumors: A Case–control Study in Sweden." Cancer Causes and Controls *4, no. 5, 465–476.*

Study author: Tynes
Date Published: 1992
Study type: Standardized incidence ratio
Reported Outcome: Positive

Tynes used a more complex and sophisticated exposure assessment method than most prior studies. Using job titles from Norway's 1960 and 1970 censuses, he grouped workers according to the presumed strength of their exposures. All told, he studied 37,945 men for the years 1961–1985.

Using the 1960 census data, men classified as electrical workers had a statistically significant increase for cancers in general and for breast cancer in particular. The investigators did not find an increase for leukemia or brain cancer. When Tynes looked at workers in electrical jobs in both 1960 and 1970, however, he did find a risk of leukemia and brain cancer. The leukemia excess occurred in radio and telegraph operators, radio and TV repairmen, and power line workers and power supply electricians. The brain tumor risk was limited to men who worked along railway lines, which often also serve as rights-of-way for transmission and distribution lines.

Tynes, T, Andersen, A, and Langmark, F (1992). "Incidence of Cancer in Norwegian Workers Potentially Exposed to Electromagnetic Fields." American Journal of Epidemiology 136: 81–88.

Study author: Sahl
Date Published: 1993
Study type: Case-control
Reported Outcome: Negative

In one of the most complicated and extensive studies done of workers to date, this research team devised a complex method of calculating EM field exposures according to job titles in conjunction with calculations based on measurements taken by meters worn by workers. This methodology has been described as "exceptional." The study was done by a scientist employed by Southern California Edison, and the workers studied all were employed by the utility.

Sahl examined the records of 36,221 men and women who worked for the utility for at least one year between 1960 and 1988. The study cases were cancer deaths from leukemia, lymphoma, and brain cancer, while the controls

(10 per case) were workers alive at the time their matched cases died. The study did not evaluate the possibility that some controls may have later developed or died of one of the types of cancers studied. Using various exposure measures, Sahl found no statistically significant associations between EM field exposures and any of the three cancer types he studied. The investigation did find a modest increase in leukemias among the cases, but the rise was not significant. The study, which is already being analyzed closely and which will very likely be repeated by other investigators, has two potential flaws. First, it is unclear whether the data factored in age, which is known to be an increasing risk factor for cancer. Second, because the study compared utility workers as both cases and controls, the mean exposure of the controls may have been higher than the mean exposures of a general population.

Sahl, JD, Kalsh, MA, and Greenland, S (1993). "Cohort and Nested Case-control Studies of Hematopoietic Cancers and Brain Cancers Among Electric Utility Workers." Epidemiology *4: 104–114.*

Study author: Swerdlow
Date Published: 1993
Study type: Proportional incidence ratio
Reported Outcome: Positive

Swerdlow found a statistically significant increase in eye cancer among electrical and electronics workers for three years out of an eight-year investigation. The study looked at deaths from eye cancer from 1968 to 1975 and used job titles taken from data filed with an eye cancer registry at the time of diagnosis.

Swerdlow, AJ (1993). "Epidemiology of Eye Cancer in Adults in England and Wales, 1962–1977." American Journal of Epidemiology *118: 294–300.*

Study author: Linet
Date Published: 1993
Study type: Standardized incidence ratio
Reported Outcome: Positive

This large-scale study of non-Hodgkin's lymphoma—a type of cancer of the lymph nodes—used the same research methods as Linet's 1988 study of leukemia (see page 184). It evaluated 4,496 non-Hodgkin's lymphoma cases between 1961 and 1979 in terms of their job classifications, which were taken from the 1960 census. The investigators calculated standardized incidence ratios that compared the rates of non-Hodgkin's lymphoma among various job categories to the expected rate. They found that working in the electrical power industry was associated with a significantly increased risk. In particular, working as an engineer or an electric power plant technician had the highest risk.

Linet, MS, Malker, HSSR, et al. (1993). "Non-Hodgkin's Lymphoma and Occupation in Sweden: A Registry-based Analysis." British Journal of Industrial Medicine *50: 79–84.*

Reproductive Effects

Study authors: Wertheimer and Leeper
Date Published: 1986
Study type: Case-control
Reported Outcome: Positive

Both electric blankets and electrically heated waterbeds produce EM fields, though the exposures are usually much higher for electric blankets. If fields can affect fetal development, you would expect to see a greater problem for winter pregnancies than for summer ones, particularly in areas where winters are colder than the norm. Colorado, where Wertheimer and Leeper work, fit this criteria, and the researchers investigated pregnancy outcomes, comparing electric blanket and heated waterbed users, on the one hand, to nonusers.

They reported a cluster of miscarriages (spontaneous abortions) between September and June for couples that used electric blankets. Couples that used either electric blankets or electrically heated waterbeds had a significantly higher miscarriage rate during the same winter period. In addition, Wertheimer and Leeper also found that babies conceived among the electric blanket users between September and June had longer gestational periods. This result was statistically significant. These babies also had a higher probability of being "slow-growing" fetuses.

Wertheimer, N and Leeper, E (1986). "Possible Effects of Electric Blankets and Heated Waterbeds on Fetal Development." Bioelectromagnetics *7: 13–22.*

Study authors: Wertheimer and Leeper
Date Published: 1988
Study type: Case-control
Reported Outcome: Positive

Following up on their 1986 study that found an association between electrically heated beds and miscarriages, Wertheimer and Leeper studied birth statistics from Eugene and Springfield, Oregon, in 1983 and 1985. These areas were chosen because a high proportion of the homes there are heated using electrical cables in the ceilings or floors. By measurements and calculations, the team estimated average in-home EM field levels of about 10 milligauss in these homes.

As in their 1986 investigation, they found statistically significant seasonal variations in miscarriage rates in homes with electric cable heating, although the rates measured over a full year were the same for homes heated with electric cables and those heated by nonelectrical methods.

Wertheimer, N and Leeper, E (1988). "Fetal Loss Associated with Two Seasonal Sources of Electromagnetic Field Exposure." American Journal of Epidemiology *v: 129 (1): 220–224.*

Study author: Savitz
Date Published: 1990
Study type: Case-control
Reported Outcome: Negative

As a follow-up to his 1988 study, Savitz focused on prenatal and childhood exposures to electric appliances, including electric blankets. His study population was drawn from the group he evaluated in the earlier investigation using essentially the same EM field exposure methods.

Children who were exposed in utero to electric blanket fields were more likely to develop brain cancer and leukemia, particularly when the exposure occurred during the first trimester of the pregnancy. These findings were statistically significant. Though the number of exposed cases was small, children exposed in utero to EM fields from other suspected sources, such as electric heating pads, heated waterbeds, and electric clocks, were not at a significantly increased risk of cancer.

Savitz, DA, John, EM, Kleckner, RC (1990). "Magnetic Field Exposure from Electric Appliances and Childhood Cancer." American Journal of Epidemiology *131: 763–773.*

Study author: Sanjose
Date Published: 1991
Study type: Cohort
Reported Outcome: Positive

This study looked at the effect of parental occupation on gestation and birth among Scottish families. Women who worked at electrical jobs had an increased risk of delivering babies either prematurely or with a low birth weight. Fathers who worked in electrical occupations were not found to have affected either of these outcomes.

Sanjose, S, Roman, E, and Beral, V (1991). "Low Birth Weight and Preterm Delivery, Scotland, 1981–1984: Effects of Parents' Occupation." Lancet, 338: 428–431.

Study author: Lindbohm
Date Released: 1992
Study type: Case-control
Reported Outcome: Positive

This Finnish team found that women exposed to more than 3 milligauss EM fields from VDTs experienced more than three times the rate of miscarriages compared to women exposed to less than 3 milligauss. The finding was statistically significant. Lindbohm's team also reported that time of exposure did not associate with an increased risk, and that exposure to strong EM radiation in the very low frequency range also increased the miscarriage rate, though not significantly. VDTs that produce EM fields in excess of 3 milligauss are the exception, though they are not unheard of. New VDTs that meet the Swedish emissions guidelines emit far lower levels.

Lindbohm, ML, et al. (1992). "Magnetic Fields of Video Display Terminals and Spontaneous Abortions." American Journal of Epidemiology 136: no. 9: 1041–1051.

EM Radiation Studies

In contrast to the number of epidemiological studies of EM field exposures, EM radiation exposures are largely unstudied. This is in large part a result of the difficulty of identifying a large and reliable study population.

Cancer

Study author: Szmigielski
Date Published: 1987
Study type: Case-control
Reported Outcome: Positive

Szmigielski's team studied cancer incidence in Polish military personnel by evaluating their EM radiation and, to a lesser extent, their EM field exposures. They found "large and consistent differences" in cancer rates, particularly for cancers of the blood and the lymph nodes. They also found a significant increase in cancer incidence for all types of cancer combined. In an earlier study, Szmigielski reported that exposed military personnel developed cancer at three times the rate of nonexposed personnel.

Szmigielski, S, et al. (1987). Cited in *Evaluation of the Potential Carcinogencity of Electromagnetic Fields. Washington, D.C.:* Environmental Protection Agency *(1990), 3–17–3–72.*

Study author: Garaj-Vrhovac
Date Published: 1992
Study type: Uncertain
Reported Outcome: Positive

This Croation team has reported that radar maintenance workers experienced unusual changes in their eyes, blood, and brain over several years of regular exposure. The researchers identified chromosomal changes they linked to the effects. The findings are notable because a parallel study done in the laboratory has found similar chromosomal changes in exposed cells. During the human study, the researchers observed chromosomal changes in the workers after they were exposed to very high EM radiation levels from one of the air traffic control radars they worked on.

Garaj-Vrhovoc, V, Aleksandra, F, and Durda, H (1992). "A Mutagenic Study Among Radar Station Personnel" (abstract). Proceedings of the 1st Congress of the European Bioelectromagnetics Assocation, *January 23–25, 1992.*

Goldoni, J, and Djurek, M (1992). "Health Status of Personnel Occupationally Exposed to Microwaves and Radiofrequencies" (abstract). Proceedings of the 1st Congress of the European Bioelectromagnetics Assocation, *January 23–25, 1992.*

Reproductive Effects

Reported clusters of miscarriages and fetal malformations among women using computers, or video display terminals (VDTs), spurred a series of studies in the 1980s. Because VDTs emit a little-studied type of EM radiation in the very low frequency, or VLF, range, and because there was no other apparent reason for computer work to cause reproductive problems, the studies assumed they were testing whether EM radiation adversely affected pregnancy or fetal development. Here are the major studies.

Study author: McDonald
Date Published: 1986
Study type: Case-control
Reported Outcome: Negative

McDonald found a statistically significant increase in miscarriages among women who used video display terminals, or VDTs, but she concluded that the finding was caused by flaws in the study methodology.

This study evaluated 17,632 pregnancies among women working with VDTs between 1982 and 1984. It was part of a larger study of 100,000 women in Montreal, Quebec,

Canada, during that period. McDonald's team found that women who used VDTs seven to twenty-nine hours per week had the greatest increased risk among VDT users. Overall, the investigators concluded that the observed excess was due to the difficulty study participants could have had in recalling key details that occurred several years earlier, a factor known as recall bias. Other scientists questioned the validity of this assessment and suggested that McDonald's study was, in fact, positive.

McDonald, AD, Cherry, NM, Delorme, C, and McDonald, JC (1986). "Visual Display Units and Pregnancy: Evidence from the Montreal Survey." Journal of Occupational Medicine 28: no. 12: 1226–1231.

Study author: Goldhaber
Date Published: 1988
Study type: Case-control
Reported Outcome: Positive

This study of 1,583 pregnancies among women who used video display terminals, or VDTs, in 1981 and 1982 was one of the first on this type of EM radiation exposure. Throughout the first half of the 1980s, reports of clusters of both miscarriages and fetal defects among VDT operators stirred general concern about emissions. By their nature, clusters—an apparently increased number of, in this case, reproductive problems among a small group of women—are difficult to interpret. Clusters often occur by chance, but a large number of clusters may indicate a problem. The next logical step to reported clusters is an epidemiological study such as this one.

Goldhaber's team found that women who worked at VDTs more than twenty hours per week were significantly more likely to have miscarriages compared to women whose jobs were similar but who did not use VDTs. Comparing the VDT workers to nonworking women, the increase in miscarriages was even greater. A subgroup of the twenty-plus-hour VDT users—administrative support and clerical workers—had the highest risk found in the experiment compared to workers in comparable job categories who did not operate computers. This subgroup also had a dose–response relationship between the number of hours at a computer and the miscarriage risk. Women who used VDTs fewer than twenty hours per week did not have a significantly increased risk.

The study found too few cases to analyze whether the VDT users faced an increased risk for birth defects, although they did identify a nonsignificant increase among VDT operators who used the machines at least five hours per week. The research team did not attempt to take EM radiation measurements, and they explained the problems inherent in using VDT use as a surrogate for exposure:

> Exposure itself is imperfectly measured by time spent working on the machines. The highest [EM radiation] emissions are from the back, sides, and even tops of the machine, not the front. Exposure can be dependent on office seating arrangements and coworkers' use of the machines.

They explained, however, that this makes it likely that their results understate the extent of the miscarriage problem. They also noted in their published report that the results may reflect other factors, such as stress and ergonomic factors. In addition, this study may have been influenced by recall bias.

Goldhaber, MK, Polen, MR, and Hiatt, RA (1988). "The Risk of Miscarriage and Birth Defects Among Women Who Use Visual Display Terminals During Pregnancy." American Journal of Industrial Medicine 13: 695–706.

Study authors: Nurminen and Kurppa
Date Published: 1988
Study type: Case-control
Reported Outcome: Negative

This evaluation of 1,044 women found no significant differences among VDT users, non-VDT–using office workers, and women who did not work in offices, but serious methodological shortcomings limit the usefulness of the conclusion. Nurminen and Kurppa reported no differences in birth weights, weights of the placentas, duration of gestation, and reported symptoms of spontaneous abortion among the three groups. Women who had spontaneous abortions and who gave birth to babies with defects were not included in the study population, however. EM radiation exposures were estimated on the basis of job titles and the women's descriptions of the work.

Nurminen, T and Kurppa K (1988). "Office Employment, Work with Video Display Terminals, and Course of Pregnancy." Scandinavian Journal of Work and Environmental Health *14, no. 5: 293–298.*

Study author: Schnorr
Date Published: 1991
Study type: Case-control
Reported Outcome: Negative

Working out of the National Institute for Occupational Safety and Health, Schnorr's team used a questionable method to conclude that VDT emissions—both EM field and EM radiation—did not increase the miscarriage rate among women using VDTs compared to women using other types of displays.

The study relied on a comprehensive set of EM field and EM radiation measurements made more than eighteen months after interviews for the study were done. The measurements showed wide variation in EM radiation emissions among seemingly identical VDTs, but these differences were not factored into Schnorr's analysis. In addition, the measurements showed that cases and controls were exposed to the same EM field levels, preventing meaningful comparisons. The study involved interviews with some 2,400 women who worked as telephone operators using either traditional VDTs (the cases) or other displays that did not contain EM radiation-emitting devices.

Schnorr, T, et al. (1991). "Video Display Terminals and the Risk of Spontaneous Abortion." New England Journal of Medicine 324: 727–733.

APPENDIX B

An EM Field
and EM
Radiation Primer

EM FIELDS AND EM RADIATION ARE FORMS OF ELECTROMAGNETIC energy, similar in many ways to visible light, X rays, ultraviolet radiation, and other forms of electromagnetic energy. For the purpose of evaluating health risks, they are different, however, for reasons explained later. All forms of electromagnetic energy are classified on a continuum known as the electromagnetic energy spectrum (see Table 4).

The spectrum is divided into two parts—nonionizing electromagnetic energy and ionizing electromagnetic energy. Ionizing energy such as X rays is strong enough to destabilize a molecule by changing its structure. Nonionizing energy can affect a molecule in a variety of ways, but it does not change its basic structure.

Energy in the nonionizing range is most readily understood as waves—sort of like ocean waves and sound waves. The waves have certain characteristics such as frequency, wavelength, amplitude, and wave shape that allow us to describe them and explain how they work. Figure 5 describes some of these characteristics.

TABLE 4

The Electromagnetic Energy Spectrum

Nonionizing electromagnetic energy
Direct current (DC)
Extremely low frequency (ELF), also known as power
   frequency
Very low frequency
Radiofrequency
   Long wave
   Medium wave
   Short wave
   Very high frequency (TV)
   Ultra high frequency (TV)
Microwaves
Infrared radiation
Visible light
Ultraviolet radiation

Ionizing electromagnetic energy
   X rays
   Gamma rays

Figure 5

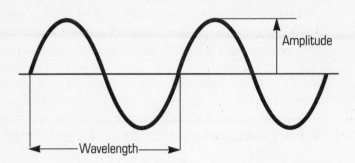

Amplitude

Wavelength

This wave illustrates the changing strength, or *amplitude*, of electromagnetic energy over distance. As the strength increases and the energy travels, the wave rises and moves to the right. As the strength decreases and time passes, the wave declines and moves to the right. Strength is shown on the vertical axis (up and down) and distance is shown on the horizontal axis (from left to right), as shown below.

Figure 6

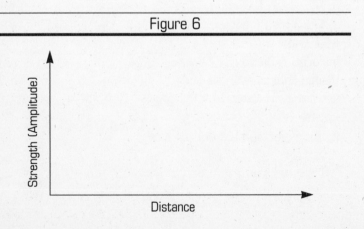

Strength (Amplitude)

Distance

Frequency

On the spectrum, energy is organized by *frequency*, with direct current having the lowest frequency (0) and gamma rays having the highest. The frequency of a wave is the number of times per second that a complete wave (or one wavelength) passes a fixed point. The electricity we use to light our homes and operate our TV sets has a frequency of 60 cycles per second. The scientific term for cycles per second is *hertz*, abbreviated Hz. By comparison, microwaves range in the millions to billions of hertz.

Power frequency is 60 Hz in the United States but 50 Hz in most other industrialized nations. Both fall into the extremely low frequency (below 3,000 hertz), or ELF, range on the electromagnetic spectrum (see Figure 7). EM radiation includes the frequencies above extremely low frequency up to visible light. As the following illustration shows, this includes many energy forms.

Wavelength

Wavelength is another key wave characteristic. It is the distance from the starting point of one wave to the starting point of the next wave. As a wave's frequency increases, its wavelength decreases, and vice versa. At 60 Hz, the wavelength is about 3,100 miles. At radiofrequency ranges, the wavelength is closer to thirty or forty feet, and at microwave ranges it is approximately one inch.

Amplitude

Wave *amplitude* is the height of the wave from the middle of the top-to-bottom wave cycle. Amplitude tells you the strength

Figure 7

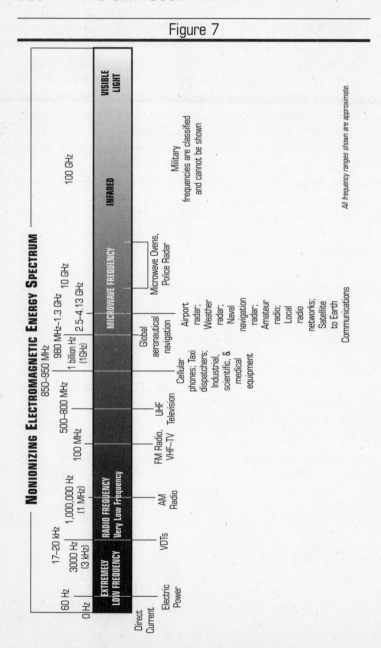

NONIONIZING ELECTROMAGNETIC ENERGY SPECTRUM

All frequency ranges shown are approximate.

of the field. Amplitude can and does vary considerably without changing frequency or wavelength. That is, a 60 Hz wave can have an amplitude of 10 or an amplitude of 10,000.

Not all waves are alike. The wave shown on page 218 is a simple illustration known as a *sine* wave. In reality, waves have an infinite number of shapes. This is important because research suggests that wave shape may play a key role in causing biological effects. The speed with which waves reach their maximum amplitude and the speed at which they return to zero seems to influence how EM fields and EM radiation affect people and other living things. Researchers are particularly interested in knowing more about waves that reach their peak amplitudes very quickly—known as pulsed EMFs, or pulsed EM radiation.

ELECTRICAL CHARGES

EM fields and EM radiation are the products of electrical *charges*—minuscule particles that are the building blocks of the physical world. Charges can be negative or positive, and all charges produce effects on—or interact with—other, nearby charges. Opposite charges attract each other and similar charges repel each other. When you try to push together the positive ends of two different magnets, you physically experience charges repelling one another.

CURRENT

Electrical charges flowing through a wire or another conductor are known as electric *current*. When an electric blanket is plugged in but turned off, the electric charges are stationary. When you turn it on, the charges flow as current.

Everywhere there is electrical current there is a magnetic field. Magnetic fields, in turn, create electric fields by a process called *induction*. The two types of fields combined are the EM field.

Current is most easily conveyed through conductors such as wires (insulators are, by definition, poor conductors). A conductor in an EM field can experience magnetic induction—in effect, the creation of a current on the conductor as a result of its interaction with the field. The human body is a conductor, so EM fields induce electric currents in our bodies.

FIELDS

A *field* is the area in which charges interact with other charges. Most people find it difficult to visualize a field, but once you can you will find it much easier to understand this topic.

Imagine the earth as a charged particle. The area in space in which the earth's gravity affects the movement of other objects is the earth's gravitational field. The moon is in the field, and so its orbit is affected by it. Pluto, for practical purposes, is outside of the field. Now, consider the complexity of fields interacting in the entire universe. In our physical world there are a virtually infinite number of charged particles interacting with one another.

Charges can be either stationary or moving. When the charged particles are still, they produce an *electric field* that interacts only with other stationary charges. The strength of the electric field is determined by the amount of the charge. Charge is measured in volts, so a high-voltage power line creates a stronger electric field than does a low-voltage line.

When charges are moving, they interact only with other

moving charges. This is the *magnetic field*. The strength of the magnetic field is determined by the amount of current, measured in amperes, or amps. A power line delivering electricity to a group of homes all of which are running air conditioners—and so are drawing large amounts of current—produces a stronger magnetic field than a power line providing electricity to a set of vacant houses. Remember this crucial fact: *stationary charges produce electric fields; moving charges produce magnetic fields.*

Health researchers believe that the magnetic field component is more likely to be associated with health hazards and so they are interested primarily in flowing charges (current).

FIELD DIRECTION

Electric and magnetic fields related to a single source—for example, a single wire—propagate at right angles to one another. If the magnetic field is parallel to the ground, the electric field is perpendicular to the ground. The exact orientation is determined by the direction the electromagnetic wave is moving, as shown in Figure 8.

EM RADIATION

The key differences between EM fields and EM radiation are the amount of energy (EM radiation has more) and the frequency (EM radiation uses higher frequencies, hence shorter wavelengths). This means that EM radiation can travel farther and so is more useful for applications such as TV and radio broadcasts.

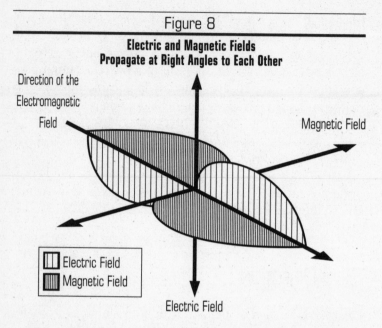

Figure 8

**Electric and Magnetic Fields
Propagate at Right Angles to Each Other**

Direction of the
Electromagnetic
Field

Magnetic Field

Electric Field

Electric Field
Magnetic Field

Like EM fields, EM radiation is produced by charges. When charges are accelerating, a force known as *electromagnetic resistance* produces EM radiation. Engineers have learned how to control the acceleration to produce a large number of EM radiation signals that can carry information in forms such as cellular phone calls. Where EM fields interact only with charged particles that are nearby, EM radiation's higher energy content gives it the ability to interact with particles and objects at great distance. Radio broadcast signals are a form of EM radiation that are used precisely because they travel well (they carry the information your TV needs). Visible light is another example.

Generally, when we talk about EM fields we are interested in areas very near to an emitting source such as a toaster or a power line. When we talk about EM radiation, we are thinking of areas at relatively greater distances from the emitting source.

Heating

A microwave oven uses a type of EM radiation to heat. Because the wavelength of microwave radiation is small (less than 1 inch), it transfers energy to objects relatively efficiently. In a microwave oven, this energy transfer causes food to heat. The ability to heat is crucial to the debate over EM fields and EM radiation. EM radiation will heat objects beginning at certain amplitudes and will not heat objects at lower amplitudes. All power frequency EM fields lack the energy content to cause heating, however.

Virtually all health-based standards that have been established for EM radiation (there are none for EM fields) assume that the only known health effects result from heating. While this once seemed sensible, research as far back as the 1940s has shown health effects in animals that do not appear to be caused by heating but by some other, nonthermal or athermal, interaction. Critics of the EM field and EM radiation health effects research often contend that nonthermal effects are inconsistent with known physical facts.

Addition and Subtraction

EM fields influence other EM fields, and EM radiation influences other EM radiation. When the peaks of two waves are synchronized—that is, when they reach their maximum amplitudes at the same time—they combine to produce an amplitude equal to their sum. It is possible, for instance, for two power lines running along the same transmission towers to produce a stronger EM field than either of the two lines produce alone. This phenomenon can significantly influence exposure levels.

EM fields can subtract as well as add. When the peak

amplitude of one field is in synch with the trough (the low point) of a second field of equal strength, the net EM field is zero. In other words, EM fields can cancel one another out, a phenomenon that is particularly important in efforts to reduce emissions.

SHIELDING

Electric fields at all frequencies are easily blocked, or shielded, by conductive materials. A grounded metal object will efficiently mitigate an electric field. Trees, houses, and other objects also help reduce the strength of electric fields.

Magnetic fields are a different matter, since only specialized (and relatively expensive) metals can decrease the strength of magnetic fields. In practical terms, magnetic fields pass through almost everything. They can not easily be shielded. EM radiation, by contrast, is easily shielded. Because it has much shorter wavelengths, it is easily absorbed by most living and inanimate objects.

GLOSSARY

Alternating current (AC)   Electric current that reverses direction with a constant or regular frequency.

Ampere, or amp (A)   The unit of measure for electric current.

Cancer   The general term for malignant growths, or tumors, or for cells that grow uncontrolled. There are approximately 150 types of cancer.

Cancer initiator   An agent that can start the process by which normal cells turn into cancerous ones. Ionizing radiation and some chemicals are known initiators. The development of cancer is a multistage process that begins with initiation. Some initiated cancerous cells never develop into full-blown cancer.

Cancer promoter   An agent that aids or accelerates the development or growth of cancerous cells.

Charge   A physical property of elementary particles that causes them either to move toward (attract) or away from (repel) one another. A charge is either positive (proton) or negative (electron). The flow of charged particles is an electrical current.

Circadian rhythm A twenty-four-hour period as it pertains to behavioral or biological functions—for example, sleep.

Conduction The movement of an electrical charge through an object or substance within an electromagnetic field.

Current The organized flow of electric charges through a conductor measured in amperes. The current at a given cross section is the rate of flow. A common analogy is water flowing through a hose.

Direct current (DC) A type of current in which the flow of charges is in one direction only. Most batteries are direct current; most electric power systems are alternating current.

Distribution line A power line, often strung on telephone poles in suburban neighborhoods, used to distribute electric power to a community. Most distribution lines operate at much lower voltages than do transmission lines. The current on distribution lines, measured in amperes, often is approximately the same as that on transmission lines, however.

DNA (Deoxyribonucleic acid) The basic genetic material of humans and most living things. When cells replicate themselves, as they do constantly, the DNA also replicates itself into identical twins, one of which stays with the existing cell while the other becomes the DNA of the new cell. This process is known as DNA transcription.

Dose The amount of an exposure that produces a discernible effect. For EM fields and EM radiation, it is not clear what aspect of exposure—duration, amount, or frequency—is the key dose.

Electricity Physical phenomena related to the interaction of electric charges.

Electric field The area in which an electric charge is affected by other electric charges. The electric field strength or intensity is expressed scientifically by the symbol E.

Electric power The rate of energy use or work in an electrical system.

Electromagnetic field (EM field) The area in the vicinity of a current-carrying electrical conductor or an electrical charge where other charges are affected.

Electromagnetic radiation (EM radiation) Energy that results when an electric charge accelerates. EM radiation (also nonionizing electromagnetic radiation or nonionizing radiation) is thought of as waves propagated through space. The electric and magnetic fields are at right angles to each other, and both are at right angles to the direction of propagation. In a vacuum, EM radiation travels at the speed of light.

Epidemiological study A type of research study that evaluates health-related factors across a relatively large human population. Epidemiological studies often rely on compiled statistical data on disease (morbidity) and death (mortality) for purposes of comparison.

Extremely low frequency (ELF) Electromagnetic energy in the approximate frequency range of 1 hertz to 3,000 hertz. ELF includes 60 hertz electric power, also referred to as power frequency.

Frequency (f) The rate at which a wave completes one full cycle. The rate per second is expressed in hertz (Hz).

Gauss (G) The unit of measure for the strength and direction of a magnetic field (magnetic flux density). Most magnetic field exposures are on the order of one one-thousandth gauss to ten one-thousandths gauss, or 1–10 milligauss.

Gauss meter A device used to measure magnetic fields.

Giga The prefix indicating one billion times a value. For example, 1 gigahertz (GHz) = 1,000,000,000 hertz.

Hertz (Hz) The unit of measure for frequency. One hertz (1 Hz) equals one cycle per second.

Hormone A chemical substance produced in one organ or body part that initiates or regulates the activity of a different group of cells or organs elsewhere in the body.

Impedance (Z) An electrical circuit's resistance to passage of a current, a key factor in determining the current's amplitude.

Induction Production of a current in a conductor by an electromagnetic field.

Kilo The prefix indicating 1,000 times a value. For example, 1 kilovolt (kV) = 1,000 volts.

Kilovolt (kV) The unit commonly used to describe electric potential of residential and commercial electrical power delivery systems. For example, while most household electricity is at 115 volts or 230 volts, transmission lines usually carry between 69 and 765 kilovolts. One kilovolt (kV) = 1,000 volts.

Kilovolt per meter (kV/m) The strength of electric fields is measured in volts per meter. Since 1 kilovolt equals 1,000 volts, "kilovolts per meter" is a commonly used description of electric field strength.

Magnetic field (H) The area in which a moving charged particle is affected by the movement of other charged particles. Magnetic field strength is expressed scientifically by the symbol H. See also *Magnetic flux density*.

Magnetic flux density The measurement of the strength and direction of a magnetic field. It is expressed scientifically by the symbol B.

Melatonin A hormone that helps the human body discern night and day. Produced by the pineal gland, it is present in larger quantities at night and in smaller quantities during the day. Melatonin also plays a role in regulating the growth of cancer cells.

Micro (μ) The prefix indicating a one-millionth part of something. For example, 1 microgauss (μG) = 1/1,000,000 gauss.

Microwaves (MW) Electromagnetic waves in the approximate frequency range of 1–300 billion hertz, or gigahertz (GHz). This is a higher frequency range than radiofrequency radiation but a lower range than infrared and visible light. Strong microwaves can cause heating in human tissue.

Milli (m) The prefix indicating a one-thousandth part of something. For example, 1 milligauss (mG) = 1/1,000 gauss.

Nonionizing electromagnetic radiation The range of the electromagnetic spectrum comprising direct current, extremely low frequencies, very low frequencies, radiofrequencies, microwaves, infrared, and visible light. Sometimes referred to by its acronym NIER, it is unlike ionizing radiation in its inability to break chemical and electrical bonds of an atom or group of atoms to lose or gain one or more electrons. X rays are one example of ionizing radiation; radio broadcasts are an example of NIER.

Nonthermal Unrelated to heat. Biological effects associated with EM fields and some EM radiation exposures are athermal, and the precise mechanisms producing the effects are unknown.

Phase The timing of an alternating current, voltage, or field.

Pineal gland Located in the brain, the pineal gland produces melatonin, a hormone that may be affected by exposure to electromagnetic fields.

Power density The amount of power—or the rate at which energy is transferred—per unit area, usually given as a form of watts per square meter (W/m^2). You most often see it as milliwatts per square centimeter (mW/cm^2), since that is the typical range of human exposures.

Radiation Energy propagated through space either as particles or as waves. See also *nonionizing radiation*.

Radiofrequency (RF) Electromagnetic energy in the approximate frequency range of 3,000 hertz (3 kHz) to 1 billion hertz (1 GHz).

RNA (Ribonucleic acid) Chemical compounds in cells made from DNA and used to carry information and materials that cells use to make proteins.

Root mean square value (RMS) A representative value of a continuously varying quantity, such as an EM field. RMS values are derived from numerous samples taken regularly during a given cycle.

Specific absorption rate (SAR) The rate at which energy is absorbed. SAR is used to describe EM radiation interactions with the body.

Stray voltage Excess electric charge returning to the transmission or distribution system, usually through the ground. Electric power distribution systems allow some unused current that goes into a home or business to return to the system via ground current—that is, electricity sent to ground (literally, into the ground) seeks to find its way back to an electric power source such as a transmission line. In some instances, most often on farms where transmission lines cross the property, this current creates electric current on metal equipment such as feeding bins for cows and other animals. When this happens, the animals can receive shocks sufficiently strong to change their behavior.

Tesla (T) A unit once commonly used to measure magnetic fields. Because 1 tesla is a large quantity in the context of the current health debate, most scientists use the gauss unit instead; 1 tesla = 10,000 gauss = 10 million milligauss.

Transmission line The electric power lines used to carry large amounts of electric power long distances. Most transmission lines operate between 69 and 765 kilovolts, using three-phase power systems. Transmission lines commonly are carried along large metal towers.

Very low frequency (VLF)   Electromagnetic energy in the approximate frequency range of 3,000 hertz (3 kHz) to 30,000 hertz (30 kHz).

Volt (V)   The unit used to measure electrical potential.

Watt (W)   The unit used to measure electric power.

Wave   A regular, periodic disturbance in space. In electricity and for EM fields and EM radiation, the disturbances (the electric and magnetic fields) are at right angles to the direction the wave is traveling. The main characteristics of a wave are the speed it is traveling, its frequency, its wavelength, and its amplitude. The wavelength is equal to the speed of propagation divided by the frequency.

Wavelength   The distance between comparable points of two successive waves.

X rays or X radiation   A common type of ionizing radiation.

FURTHER READING

This list includes documents that will add to your under-standing of the medical, historical, and political facets of EM fields and EM radiation. Citations for selected published epidemiological research are in Appendix A.

BOOKS AND ARTICLES

Becker, M. D., O. Robert, and Gary Selden. *The Body Electric: Electromagnetism and the Foundation of Life.* New York: William Morrow, 1985.

Brodeur, Paul. *The Zapping of America: Microwaves, Their Deadly Risk, and the Cover-Up.* New York: W.W. Norton & Co., 1977.

———. *The Great Power-Line Cover-Up: How the Utilities and the Government Are Trying to Hide the Cancer Haz-*

ards Posed by Electromagnetic Fields. Boston: Little, Brown, 1993.

————. *Currents of Death: Power Lines, Computer Terminals, and the Attempt to Cover Up Their Threat to Your Health*. New York: Simon & Schuster, 1989.

Bierbaum, Philip J., and John M. Peters. *Proceedings of the Scientific Workshop on the Health Effects of Electric and Magnetic Fields on Workers: January 30–31, 1991*. Cincinnati, OH: National Institute for Occupational Safety and Health, 1991.

Environmental Protection Agency. "Evaluation of the Potential Carcinogenicity of Electromagnetic Fields" (Review Draft), EPA 600/6–90/005B, 1990.

————. "EMF in Your Environment: Magnetic Field Measurements of Everyday Electrical Devices," Report 402–R–92–008, December 1992.

————. "Questions and Answers About Electric and Magnetic Fields (EMFs)," Report 402–R–92–009, December 1992.

EMF Information Project. "EMF Issue in Sweden: Trip Report, March 16–24, 1993," Report Number 9303FS3, undated.

Florig, H. Keith. "Mitigation of Electromagnetic Field Exposure in Offices," Resources for the Future, Washington, DC, October 1991.

————. "Containing the Costs of the EMF Problem." *Science* 257 (July 24, 1992), pp. 468–492.

McCune, Philip S. "The Power Line Health Controversy: Legal Problems and Proposals for Reform." *University of Michigan Law Journal of Law Reform* 24: 1.

Morgan, M. Granger. "Electric and Magnetic Fields from 60 Hertz Electric Power: What Do We Know About Possible Health Risks." Carnegie Mellon University, Pittsburgh, PA, 1989.

————. "Measuring Power Frequency Fields." Carnegie Mellon University, Pittsburgh, PA, 1992.

————. "What Can We Conclude from Measurements of Power Frequency Fields." Carnegie Mellon University, Pittsburgh, PA, 1993.

Moore, Taylor. "Exploring the Options for Magnetic Field Management." *EPRI Journal* (October/November 1990): 5–19.

Nair, Indira, M. Granger Morgan, and H. Keith Florig. "Biological Effects of Power Frequency Electric and Magnetic Fields." Background Paper, U.S. Congress, Office of Technology Assessment (OTA–BP–E–53), May 1989.

New York State Power Lines Project. "Biological Effects of Power Line Fields." Albany, NY, 1987.

Sagan, Leonard. "Epidemiological and Laboratory Studies of Power Frequency Electric and Magnetic Fields." *Journal of the American Medical Association* 268, no. 5 (August 5, 1992): 625–629.

Silva, Mike, Norm Hummon, David Rutter, and Chris Hooper. "Power Frequency Magnetic Fields in the Home." Paper presented at the IEEE/PES 1988 Winter Meeting, New York City, January 31–February 5, 1988.

Steneck, Nicholas H. *The Microwave Debate*. Cambridge, MA: MIT Press, 1984.

U.S. Congress. "Electric Powerlines: Health and Public Policy Implications. Oversight Hearing before the Subcommittee on General Oversight and Investigation, Committee on Interior and Insular Affairs; U.S. House of Representatives, 101st Congress: Second Session, March 8, 1990." Washington, DC: U.S. Government Printing Office, 1990.

————. "EMF and High-Voltage Power Lines: A Case Study in Michigan. Hearings before the Subcommittee on Investigations and Oversight of the Committee on Sci-

ence, Space, and Technology; U.S. House of Representatives, 102nd Congress: First Session, August 6, 1991." Washington, DC: U.S. Government Printing Office, 1991.
————. "National Electromagnetic Fields Research and Public Information Dissemination Act: Hearing before the Subcommittee on Environment of the Committee on Science, Space, and Technology; U.S. House of Representatives, 102nd Congress: Second Session, March 10, 1992." Washington, DC: U.S. Government Printing Office, 1992.
White, Don J., Michael Barge, Eric A. George, and Karl Riley. *The EMF Controversy & Reducing Exposure from Magnetic Fields: ELF Magnetic Field Reduction from Power Utilities to Home Wiring.* Gainesville, VA: Interference Control Technologies, Inc., 1993.

Newsletters

EMF Health Report, 1500 Locust Street, Suite 3216, Philadelphia, PA 19102.
Electromagnetic Field Litigation Reporter, PO Box 1000, Westtown, PA 19395.
EMF News, 1720 I Street, NW, Suite 800, Washington, DC 20006.
Between the Lines: EMF, 83 Edison Drive, Augusta, ME 04330.
Microwave News, PO Box 1799, Grand Central Station, New York, NY 10163.

INDEX

Large Public Power Council (LPPC), 138–39
Laser printers, 17, 63–64, 66
Lawsuits, 55, 122–23, 126, 133, 143–44, 147–51
LCC (low-current configuration), 23, 161
LCDs (liquid crystal displays), 70, 108
Leal, Jocelyn, 32–33
Learning disorders, 32, 43, 119–20
LED (light-emitting diodes), 70, 108
Leeper, Ed, 21, 23, 54, 160, 197, 199; wire coding system, 23, 161–62, 164. See also Wertheimer-Leeper studies
Leukemia, 22, 24, 119, 149; fetus and electric blankets, 208; negative studies, 173, 176, 178, 181, 186; occupational studies, 174, 175, 178–90, 180, 182, 185–88, 198, 200, 201–2, 204–5; Swedish study, 166, 179; transmission lines and substations, 175–76
Liboff, Dr. Abe, 27
Lieberman, Senator Joseph, 117
Light boxes and dimmers, 64, 86
Los Angeles County, 164, 174, 179, 185
Lunde, Shirley, 141
Lung cancer, 173, 199
Lymph system cancers, 199–200, 210
Lymphocytic leukemia, 185, 203
Lymphoma, 200, 204

McLean, Dr. Jack, 30
Magnetic field: levels, 60, 73, 77, 79, 81, 163; protection in home and office, 60–72, 82–85; real estate and schools, 85–87; reducing external exposure, 72–81; shielding from, 226
Magnetic flux density (B), 230
Magnetic levitation trains, 72
Magnetic Resonance Imaging (MRI), 103–4
Magnetite, 28–29
Male breast cancer, 22, 119, 189, 190, 204; studies, 194–96
Massachusetts, 151
Mechanisms of interaction, 13, 25–34
Media, 118, 120, 121, 147–48
Medical applications, 17, 18–19, 102, 103–4
Melatonin levels, 27–28, 230
Memory loss, 32
Metal equipment, 87, 146
Metal shielding, 65, 93, 226
Michigan, 147
Microwave ovens, 11, 17, 38, 44, 89, 109, 117, 143; leakage detectors, 65, 112
Microwave phone signals, 17, 90
Microwave transmitters, 31, 97–98, 134, 144
Microwaves (MW), 219, 230
Milham, S., Jr., 178–79, 180, 182, 198, 199–200
Military, 18–19, 91, 106, 132–33
Miller, Representative George, 145
Milligauss levels, 42, 79, 145, 162, 163, 166, 176, 195, 207, 209
Minnesota, 145
Miscarriage rates, 207, 209, 211–15
Mixers, 44

Modems, wireless, 109
Modulation, 92
Monitors: baby-room, 95–96, 109, 110; medical, 103, 104
Montana, 145
Morgan, Granger, 11, 138
Mortality rates, 157
Mount Sutro, San Francisco, 99
MPR2 ("Test Methods for Visual Display Units"), 69
Mu metal inserts, 69
Multiple myelomas, 200
Municipal buildings, 81
Myelogenous leukemia, 174, 182, 186, 187, 188
Myeloid leukemia, 180, 182, 185, 199–200

National Academy of Sciences, 141
National Association of Attorneys General (NAAG), 136
National Electrical Manufacturers Association, 137
National Energy Strategy Bill (1992), 140
National Institute for Environmental Health Sciences (NIEHS), 129
National Institute for Occupational Safety and Health (NIOSH), 68, 130, 188, 214
NERP (National EM Fields Research Program), 133–34, 138, 141; and HEI model, 136; joint funding issue, 137–41; Power Line Project, 135
Nervous system. See Central nervous system
Neuroblastomas, 168, 169, 170
New Jersey, 145, 148

MARK A. PINSKY is the author of *The Carpal Tunnel Syndrome Book*, *The VDT Book: A Computer User's Guide to Health & Safety*, and *Every Citizen's Environmental Handbook*.